PAIN, DISTRESS
AND THE NEWBORN BABY

MARGARET SPARSHOTT

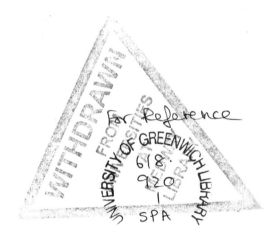

**Blackwell
Science**

© 1997 by Blackwell Science Ltd,
a Blackwell Publishing Company
Editorial Offices:
9600 Garsington Road, OX4 2DQ, UK
 Tel: +44 (0)1865 776868
Blackwell Science, Inc., 350 Main Street,
Malden, MA 02148-5018, USA
 Tel: +1 781 388 8250
Iowa State Press, a Blackwell Publishing
Company, 2121 State Avenue, Ames, Iowa
50014-8300, USA
 Tel: +1 515 292 0140
Blackwell Publishing Asia Pty Ltd,
550 Swanston Street, Carlton South,
Melbourne, Victoria 3053, Australia
 Tel: +61 (0)3 9347 0300
Blackwell Wissenschafts Verlag,
Kurfürstendamm 57, 10707 Berlin, Germany
 Tel: +49 (0)30 32 79 060

First published 1997
Reprinted 2003

Library of Congress
Cataloging-in-Publication Data

Sparshott, Margaret.
 Pain, distress, and the newborn baby/
Margaret Sparshott.
  p.   cm.
 Includes bibliographical references
and index.
 ISBN 0–632–04077–7 (alk. paper)
 1. Infants (Newborn)—Care.   I. Title.
RJ253.5.S64   1966
618.92′01—dc20   96–23903
                                CIP

ISBN 0-632-04077-7

A catalogue record for this title
is available from the British Library

Set in 10/12.5 Century Book
by DP Photosetting, Aylesbury, Bucks
Printed and bound in Great Britain by
Marston Lindsay Ross International Ltd,
Oxfordshire

For further information on
Blackwell Publishing, visit our website:
www.blackwellpublishing.com

Dedication

To 'Daniel', now a young man – wherever he may be;
and to all the Neonatal Intensive Care babies
who fight the good fight with all their might.

Contents

Contents

Foreword

Kathleen A. VandenBerg, MA
Director, Infant Development Program NICU
Stanford University School of Medicine, California

I met Ms Spashott when I was invited to England to participate in a study day for neonatal nurses in intensive care nurseries. At that time, it became clear to me that the entire country was searching for an understanding of stress and its effects on the newborn infant. I sensed a keen interest in Ms Sparshott to articulate the needs of the newborn infant in the hospital.

I believe that this work accomplishes that goal and is a very important contribution. This author not only acknowledges stress and pain in infants, but also the stress of parents and staff caring for infants in intensive care. As Ms Sparshott states: 'parents feel that they can only look on while doctors and nurses assault their babies; doctors and nurses are worried about the possible consequences of their actions, and are frustrated that they cannot do more to avoid them' (p. 159). This is a difficult truth, and Ms Sparshott honestly places this issue at the heart of the matter for all medical staff when she asks: 'does early suffering have later consequences?'. This question underlies the stress and concerns felt by all professionals who work to improve medical and developmental outcome in our high risk infant populations.

An important premise underlying this book is that unless we acknowledge infant stress, we cannot do anything about it. This book not only deals with this acknowledgement, but offers a range of behavioural and sensitive interventions for caregivers throughout. Moreover, the premise that the baby is an active partner in his care and can actively communicate to the caregivers in the interaction process, is clear. As she states 'intervention should always be dictated by the response of the baby'. In several incidences and many creative ways she gathers together the components of care which constitute comfort and consolation in an exquisitely sensitive and supportive manner.

As she deals with the issues of helplessness, fear, depression and pain in infancy, Ms Sparshott lays a foundation, first in Part I, *The Baby and the Environment* and later in Part II, *The Invasive Environment*. This discussion includes the current theory and knowledge base we have accumulated about infant behaviour, as well as a summary of current pain research. The contributions of genetics, psychoanalytic theory, central nervous system development, and the roles of memory and experiences all add to a rich review of the many perspectives which have attempted to understand infant stress and pain. By describing the types of pain and traumatic events and procedures which permeate the experience of every neonate in intensive care, Ms Sparshott sensitises us to the totality of this experience.

One of my favourite phrases in this book is 'the holding environment' (Part III) and I have already found myself using this lovely term in my own speaking. This means 'making a home' in the NICU and means here that a 'holding environment' can be made for the parents to be with their infant. In other words we need to attempt in our interactions to be 'with' infants and not do 'to' infants. What a challenge this presents! It is wonderful and refreshing to hear it proposed. Focussing on the trust that must develop between families and staff, Ms Sparshott states that a healthy relationship between family and nursery staff is essential. The involvement of the parent in the nursery experience does not just mean seeing parents as stressed visitor. It also means that staff need to take the opportunity to provide a unique experience for parents to be involved meaningfully and consistently with their infants through observation of their infant and the recording of their infant's behavioural responses. Clearly this helps parents 'to be able to take pleasure in the passing of milestones and feel that they themselves were instrumental in ... so doing' (p. 124). Research to date has shown repeatedly that bringing the parents and their infants together in a caregiving relationship can ameliorate the pain and stress for families in this situation.

Caring for the Caregivers (Chapter 10) offers an extremely important message; that is, if we acknowledge our own stress in this work, then we will acknowledge the infant's and the parent's stress. The issue for intensive care nursery staff is one of inflicting pain on a baby which seems barbaric and unnatural. In addition 'the line between what we will support day by day and what suddenly becomes unendurable is a fine one ...'. The issues for staff are not typical and the acknowledgement of staff burn out, stress related illnesses, salaries incompatible with responsibility, along with rage, frustration and anger over the moral and ethical dilemmas faced daily, working in an intensive care nursery, must be dealt with. Because, as is also noted, 'until they come to terms with their own feelings about the job, it may be difficult for nurses ... in neonatal care to understand parental attitudes and to cope with parents' feelings'. Ms Sparshott appropriately points out that, even with all the anxiety and stress and pain, nurses in this arena love their work and bring to it an 'uncompromising dedication'.

Not only can she articulate the issues for staff, but it is clear that Ms Sparshott can also imagine herself in the baby's place. She has a sensitive empathy for what the baby is feeling and offers an excellent guide for nurses to do the same. This work should be of unique interest to nurses who believe that the heart of their profession is to comfort and console in spite of the intense frustration that goes with the job.

This book leave me feeling hopeful, and relieved that there are avenues towards peace and harmony in the nursery. Of course not all outcomes will be perfect and not all staff will be happy in their jobs, but in the clear honest stating of the situation, which this work achieves, we can come to a point in which we can face each other in the nursery and say 'we can make a home in the NICU' and create 'the holding environment'.

Acknowledgements

My grateful thanks to Mary Boen, Barbara Weller and Dr Michael Quinn for agreeing to act as referees for the text; to the many friends and colleagues (too many to name) both here and overseas who have kindly sent me relevant information and articles: to Dr Harry Baumer, Sister Margaret Hunt and all my colleagues of the Neonatal Intensive Care Unit, Derriford Hospital, Plymouth for their advice and practical help over the years; to the staff of the Medical Library for the great amount of work they have done for me; and to my sister Elizabeth, for her support, encouragement and endless patience during the time it has taken to write this book.

Explanation of the Text

For the sake of clarity and simplicity, I have referred to the baby as 'he' and the caregiver as 'she' throughout; I ask the reader to understand that the text refers equally to female babies and male caregivers.

Many of the problems discussed in the book concern both the preterm and the sick term baby; I will use the term 'fragile' to describe these babies.

References to the Neonatal Unit (NU) include both the Neonatal Intensive Care Unit and the Special Care Baby Unit, unless problems specific to each are discussed.

References to 'caregivers' include all who care for the babies in the NU – doctors, nurses, midwives, parents, physiotherapists, social workers, and so on; whoever is responsible for the baby at any given moment.

References to 'nurses' include midwives, paediatric nurses, and students of different courses, caring for babies in the NU. Again, this is for simplicity – I ask members of the different professions to forgive me for not being specific.

The 'we' referred to throughout are the caregivers as described above, and as a clinical nurse I include myself in this category. I use the first person to express my own observations and experiences.

List of Abbreviations

APIB	Assessment of Preterm Infant Behavior
b.i.d.	bis in die (twice a day)
BPD	bronchopulmonary dysplasia
CMV	Continuous Mandatory Ventilation
CNS	central nervous system
CPAP	continuous positive airways pressure
DSVNI	Distress Scale for Ventilated Newborn Infants
ECMO	extra-corporeal membrane oxygenation
ET	endotracheal
g.a.	gestational age
IBCS	Infant Body Coding System
IMV	Intermittent Mandatory Ventilation
i.v.	intravenous
NACS	Neurological and Adaptive Capacity Score
NBAS	Neonatal Behavioral Assessment Scale
NEC	necrotising enterocolitis
NFCS	Neonatal Facial Coding System
NG	naso-gastric
NICU	Neonatal Intensive Care Unit
NIDCAP	Neonatal Individualized Developmental Care and Assessment Program
NIPS	Neonatal Infant Pain Score
NSAIDs	non-steroidal anti-inflammatory drugs
NU	Neonatal Unit
OG	oro-gastric
PRN	pro re nata
PTV	patient triggered ventilation
PVL	periventricular leukomalacia
q.i.d.	quater in die (four times a day)
REM	rapid-eye-movement
SCBU	Special Care Baby Unit
SHO	Senior House Officer
TAC-TIC	Touching and Caressing – Tender in Caring

List of Abbreviations

TcPO$_2$	transcutaneous oxygen
TENS	Transcutaneous Nerve Stimulation
t.i.d.	ter in die (three times a day)
TT	Therapeutic Touch
VLBW	very light birth weight

Introduction
Why a Book on Pain in Babies?

'What a little thing
To remember for years –
To remember with tears!'
William Allingham: *A Memory*

Many years ago I worked as a nurse in a unit of neonatology in Geneva. I remember one baby in particular; born at 36 weeks' g.a., he fell victim to septicaemia, resulting in hepatitis and necrotising enterocolitis. This baby (I will call him Daniel) was very ill for many weeks, requiring parenteral nutrition and long courses of antibiotics; his emaciated condition and collapsed veins made the siting of i.v. infusions increasingly difficult – soon his scalp and body were a mass of scars and contusions.

He seemed alert and responsive at birth, and at first he reacted to the constant resiting of the infusions necessary for his survival with loud, indignant crying and threshing limbs. However, after a while we noticed that Daniel no longer struggled against our hands, nor did he scream. He lay watching us in silent immobility. His eyes had developed an expression of accusation, full of a most inappropriate knowledge; Daniel had the watchful, mature look of an old man.

Daniel was so exhausted by his illness and suffering we all thought he would die – perhaps in our hearts we hoped he would; but contrary to expectations he survived. He fed vigorously, gained weight, and eventually was discharged physically well; but he remained a quiet, unresponsive baby, who neither cried nor smiled. At this time I was working at night, and never met Daniel's parents (in those days visiting hours were restricted) or discovered how they were managing to cope with seeing their child so distressed and, later, so withdrawn. Nor, since they left Switzerland soon afterwards, did we ever have news of Daniel. I often wonder what manner of man he has become.

Since then I have seen other children, for a long time subjected to repeated painful procedures, who have developed this knowing look. Not all behave with Daniel's inertia; I particularly remember two other babies who showed quite different behaviour; one continued to resist by screaming and arching her body, the other reduced response to a pitiful quiet whimpering. But common to all is the suspicious, reproachful stare.

This book was written because of the suffering of babies such as Daniel, for which I feel guilty to this day. It is the end result of a long search for anything that could help me understand the subject of pain and its effects on the newborn infant, through the exploration of books, articles, and my own memory of past experiences. The book is not only about pain, but also all the ordeals of a newborn baby in hospital. Since understanding must be followed by action, the book will also try to show how pain and distress can be relieved, and how a hostile environment can be rendered more supportive.

Pain

> 'Pain ... is a highly personal experience, depending on cultural learning, the meaning of the situation, and other factors that are unique to each individual.' (Melzack & Wall, 1988)

Pain is the response of the CNS to tissue damage, warning us from further harm by making us either reluctant to move, or quick to remove ourselves from harm's way. It comes in many forms, and is perceived by each individual in the context of his own past and present experience. The following is the definition of pain offered by Mersky in 1986, which was subsequently used by the International Association for the Study of Pain:

> 'Pain is an unpleasant sensory and emotional experience associated with actual or potential tissue damage, or described in terms of such damage.'

Note: pain is always subjective. Each individual learns the application of the word through experiences related to injury in early life. This definition combines both the physiological and psychological attributes of pain experience.

In an adult, pain perception is emotional as well as physiological. No-one truly knows the extent of another's pain, although many words have been used to describe it; words such as burning, stabbing, shooting, which draw a picture and tell a story. The newborn infant is incapable of describing sensation in such ways, since pain is a subjective experience, and babies cannot use words to tell us how they feel. Although the newborn infant is neurologically capable of sensing pain as the book will show, his intellectual and emotional perception can only be surmised; nor is he consciously aware that the discomfort he feels is due to actual damage to tissue. It could be assumed that an infant would sense pain *only* from tissue damage, as he is at the beginning of life and has no previous experience – even if learning begins in the womb, he has little information apart from the here and now – but he may feel himself to be as much traumatised by disruption as by physical intrusion (Cunningham, 1993.)

Distress

'Distress: extreme pain or suffering; that which causes suffering; calamity; exhaustion; peril; difficulty.' (*Chambers Twentieth Century Dictionary*)

Since the constantly intrusive environment of the NICU frequently provokes from the infant similar stress responses to those following a painful procedure, I have chosen to use the word distress as well as pain to indicate the way caregivers should understand such reactions. Pain can be deduced in the context of an intrusive procedure or specific illness, and the book will discuss behavioural and physiological responses to acute and chronic pain. But reactions to any form of distress will require the same techniques of comfort and consolation. If these actions are restricted to those babies who have been subjected to traumatic procedures, pain/distress due to such discomforts as hunger (after all, we talk of the 'pangs' of hunger), or the constriction of splinting, or the brightness of an overhead light may be neglected. To prevent undue suffering, caregivers must take into account every detrimental aspect of the NICU.

The newborn baby

In order to create an environment for the fragile newborn baby that will promote his well-being, it is necessary first to understand what a baby is: his capabilities; how he communicates; how he develops; what he makes of his surroundings. How is he likely to be affected by his world and the people in it? How can the behaviour of a baby be assessed, and how can he tell the caregiver he is in distress? What does he remember of early life experiences and, if these are predominantly painful, how will they affect him in the long term? What is likely to cause suffering? How can that suffering be reduced, and how can the environment be rendered more benign? How can parents cope with the stress of having a preterm or sick baby? How are the caregivers affected by their obligation to inflict pain in order to save life, and the ethical problem this presents?

In an attempt to answer these questions, the 'Model of Nursing for a Newborn Baby' based on human needs (Sparshott, 1990), which was developed from Roper's model 'Activities of Living' (1976) and the model

'Unified Whole' of Rogers (1980), can be used as a guide. Rogers emphasised the importance of the environment in the development of human potential, and this is particularly relevant to the newborn baby, who is at the beginning of life experience. According to the Model, the baby's need is 'to be cherished' and the nursing aim is 'to cherish', which means: 'to protect and treat with affection: to nurture, to nurse' (*Chambers Twentieth Century Dictionary*) – can there be a better way to describe nursing aims?

The basic physical needs of the newborn infant have been discussed in many nursing text books; the Model of Nursing for a Newborn Baby (Fig. 1) includes his emotional requirements, which are less clearly defined. The environment created for a baby must offer him security, comfort, stimulation, response to expressed needs, rest and, if all fails, the prospect of dying with dignity. I will attempt in this book to discuss all these requirements 'under one roof', and then see how they can be satisfied. Since the well-being of the baby cannot be separated from that of the parents, the parents must be involved in the attainment of these goals.

- **To be secure** – the maintenance of a safe environment. The security of the environment can be assured by attention to heat, light and sound; by the use of equipment that is well-maintained, effective but non-intrusive; by caregivers experienced in such equipment's use.
- **To be comfortable** – to be free from pain. Comfort can be provided by appropriate positioning of the baby; by understanding individual preferences; by means of pain relief and consolation techniques.
- **To develop** – to grow and to learn. Distinction needs to be made between the baby who benefits from minimal handling, and the well baby requiring stimulation.
- **To communicate** – to express needs and have them satisfied. Stress and well-being can be identified by understanding individual infant behaviour.
- **To repose** – to rest and sleep. Work can be arranged to provide the baby with periods of rest; sleep can be respected; the individual baby's state of consciousness can be taken into account when planning care.
- **To die with dignity** – encumbered only with the technical equipment that is compatible with comfort; parents and baby together in quiet, free from distraction.

During the course of the book I hope to show how a world can be created for the fragile newborn infant that will offer him positive as well as negative experiences; how the NU can become a 'home' in which he and his parents will be able to thrive. The book will explore every aspect of the NU: distress and well-being; light and sound; minimal handling and stimulation; stress among staff and parents; death; and going home.

Model of nursing based on human needs for a newborn baby within the hospital environment.
To cherish: to protect and treat with affection; to nurture, nurse (Chambers Twentieth Century Dictionary)

Nursing aims: to cherish

To deliver nursing interventions designed to satisfy these needs

To consider the baby in his own environment

To determine immediate and long-term goals for the baby and his family

To include and involve parents in the attainment of these goals

To create the most favourable environment for the development of the potential of both baby and parents

Baby's needs: to be cherished

Basic physical needs
To breathe – respiration
To be fed – nutrition
To void – elimination
To be clean – hygiene
To be warm – temperature control
To be made well – therapy

Basic emotional requirements
To be secure – the maintenance of a safe environment
To be comfortable – to be free from pain
To develop – to grow and to learn
To communicate – to express needs and have them satisfied
To repose – to rest and sleep
To die with dignity

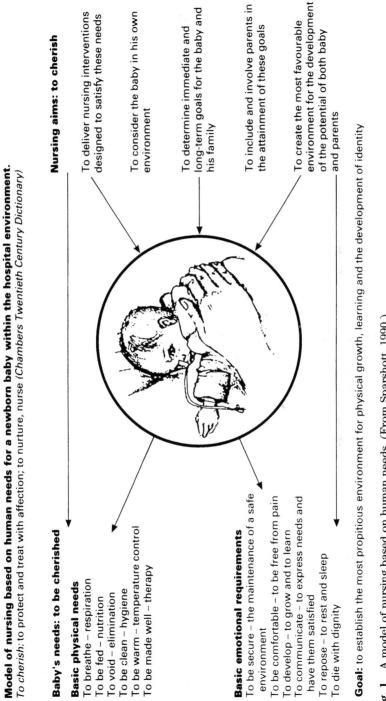

Goal: to establish the most propitious environment for physical growth, learning and the development of identity

Fig. 1 A model of nursing based on human needs. (From Sparshott, 1990.)

Is it possible to justify the trauma inflicted on babies who are unable to protest or make their own decisions? I believe that it is. The very fact that the baby is alive against such odds is in a sense a decision he has made; and with modern technology it is possible in the majority of cases to offer him not only life but also life of good quality. When the quality of life is in doubt, those involved in the care of the newborn are faced with another ethical dilemma: whether or not to continue mechanical life support. Because the burden of making such a decision weighs heavily on neonatal staff and parents, ethical problems will also be discussed in the book. But do not look for answers; answers can only be given to each particular question – and even then, very often there seems to be no right decision.

So much can be done technically to save the lives of tiny babies. I hope we as caregivers can discover some ways to make the beginning of these lives less stressful, more comfortable and more favourable for the well-being of both baby and parents.

First Memory

I remember.
I remember yes
That blissful floating
Warmth, ease,
Darkness deeply coloured,
Muffled sound,
Muffled sound.

Until I am wrenched forth
The bones of my head moulded
   together –
Agonising compression –
Tearing, forcing,
A sharp slap, and the first
Painful breath,
Bitter light without colour
And cold.
I remember the cold.

I cry, eat, sleep,
My knowledge is
A warm bed,
Arms that enfold;
Soft voices soothe, beguile –
I remember security.

Breathing tires –
Your hands demand.
Breathing pains –
Your hands command
My limbs and body, bear them down
Hands with needles probe my spine.
Hands with needles pierce my veins –
Helpless I scream into your face
Whose lines I have not learned to read;
Helpless I struggle to be freed
From hands gripping like a vice.

Now your hands are tender and kind –
Those ruthless hands that kept me
   pinned –
But I have learned to recognise
The hard and forceful hands that
   bruise
Beneath the soft hands that caress.
I feel your hands –
I remember the pain.

I look at you with the eyes
Of a wise old man;
My eyes accuse.
Could they speak
They would demand to know
Why you torment me so
Then kiss my cheek –
But memory will remain.

Memory lies deep
Where thought and knowledge sleep.

Margaret Sparshott

Part I
The Baby and the Environment

Chapter 1
The Development of Personality

Psychoanalytical terms

No discussion on the development of the individual is complete without some understanding of what is meant by 'personality'; no discussion of personality is complete without understanding certain terms, used in psychoanalysis, which identify the drives and motivations that create a person. These terms include the *psyche*, the *ego* and the *superego*.

The *psyche* is that part of the person that may be called the 'soul' or the 'mind'. It is the source of all mental and emotional life, and exists on three levels: the conscious, the subconscious and the unconscious. The *conscious* mind is aware of all that is actually happening at the present time – for instance, you are 'conscious' of reading this page. The *subconscious* consists of what is at present at the back of your mind – a taste in the mouth, the pressure of this book against your hand; these feelings are there, but will only be brought to mind when you are reminded of them. The *unconscious* is all that lies beneath present experience; memories, dreams, obscure fears, all inhabit the unconscious mind, and in certain circumstances may cause unease unless brought to the surface. The unconscious is buried memory.

The *id* is the most primitive, uninhibited, animalistic part of the personality, and is the basis of instinctive urges, mainly aggressive. It clamours for its demands to be met and, uncontrolled, will blunder on without regard for the consequences. The id represents the 'pleasure principle'. The newborn baby is almost entirely id, a mass of energies and drives needing to find a direction – maturity will bring about comparative control of the id by the development of the ego and superego.

The *ego* is the 'I' or 'self', which is compounded not only of ideas but of all forms of conscious experience, such as feelings, perception and suffering; the 'thinking self' which plans and organises and is aware of cause and effect. The *superego* lies at the other end of the scale from the id, with the ego acting as a buffer in between. The superego is 'conscience', and it is the policeman of the personality: forbidding, discouraging, counselling caution. Its prohibitions are derived from unconscious sources, such as family and social background, and conscious sources such as recent and remembered experiences. If the id represents what we would like to be, the superego represents what we ought to be, and the ego is what we are.

The ego, then, is constantly being bombarded from different sources; from the id which demands action, no matter how violent; from the superego which forbids and discourages; and from the environment which may play a positive or negative role – but which is invariably stimulating, whether for good or ill. To cope with these conflicts the ego develops certain techniques which are referred to as *ego defence mechanisms*; they are common to us all but are usually adopted only in situations of stress. The only one of these mechanisms discussed here will be *regression*, as this is central to all developmental theories (Lowe, 1972).

By 'regression' we mean the reversion of an individual to immature behaviour – the behaviour of the wife who, exasperated by her husband, throws a vase at him. She allows her id to get the better of her superego and behaves instinctively, as she would have done when she was an infant and her ego had not yet developed. It is quite natural for people to react in this way from time to time when stressed. Most people, however, would only throw the vase if it was a souvenir from the seaside, and would leave the Ming unbroken. It is the immature personality that destroys without counting the cost.

Regression is a reaction of the ego to a 'fault' or 'failure' in the environment occurring at an early age – this can be a failure in the sense of either overgratification or insufficient satisfaction. Regression is not always detrimental; a horse refusing a jump may clear it next time by going back a short way and starting again. It becomes a serious condition only when the adult returns to childhood and remains there, unable to cope with the existing world.

Another term frequently used in connection with the development of the personality is *narcissism*; overwhelming self-love. The term narcissistic is sometimes used to describe the complete self-absorption of the newborn baby, who at the beginning cannot separate the world from himself; he only comes to perceive himself as a separate being over a period of time.

Pre-natal existence

At one time it was believed that babies were 'clean slates', having no past experience, traditional values, or social consciousness to guide them as to how to behave. It was thought that they were passive receptors of outside experience, with no control over their immediate environment:

'the unitary reality of paradise prevails in the early post-natal situation' (Neumann, 1973). The earliest phase in the development of the individual is known as *paradisiacal*, since it is normally a time of comfort, security and ease. All the foetus has to do is grow; the mother is the source of all that is necessary for this purpose, and is a shield against the outside world (Wolke, 1987). At this stage the foetus has no sense of self. It seems likely, however, that an attempt may well be made by the foetus to comprehend the uterine environment, even if birth is still assumed by many to be the time for learning to begin; this pre-ego phase of existence, although known to us only in the most shadowy of experiences, is of crucial importance to the individual (Neumann, 1973).

The concept of an infant in a paradisiacal state is an attractive one to contemplate from a distance in time. It is reassuring to believe that for the unborn baby all things are perfect – perfect harmony, a blissful suspension, no pain or discomfort. This does not seem to be the case, however; experience and learning, as well as growth, are there from conception, body and psyche developing together.

Developmental theories

It is impossible for caregivers to know what it is like to be a baby; subconsciously we may 'remember' our infancy, but our conscious minds can only conjecture. The 'psychology' of infants can only be inferred, but these inferences have led to certain theories being proposed which each concentrate on a different aspect of development, focusing on internal or external influences.

Biological theorists emphasise internal and biological influences such as genetic programming and heredity as playing the most powerful role in the development of the personality. *Maturation*, which is the 'developmental process leading to the state of maturity' (Reber, 1985), comes about as the body undergoes a sequence of physical changes, such as in size and shape and hormonal patterns, and these sequential patterns of change are both common to the human species in general, and unique to each individual, dependent on the instructions passed on by the genetic and hereditary background.

Biological theorists do not exclude the influence of environment on behaviour, but they believe that the child is 'born' with characteristic patterns of responding to the environment and to the people who compose it; in other words, a child is born with a distinct 'temperament', and this inherent temperament modifies the way in which he responds to the world about him, and the way in which that world responds to him.

Learning is the process by which knowledge is acquired through reinforced practice. *Learning theorists* acknowledge the importance of biological factors in development, but maintain that the individual behaviour of the child is determined by his observation and learning of the environment.

Cognition is the mental process by which knowledge is acquired, and can broadly be taken to include thinking, problem solving and reasoning. *Cognitive-developmental theorists* see the child's ability to adapt to the world about him as playing the key role in the formation of personality. The original emphasis was on the development of thinking (hence 'cognitive-developmental') but the same fundamental ideas and assumptions have been applied to social and emotional development.

Psychoanalytical theorists emphasise both the internal qualities of the child and the external influences of the environment. They seek to explain human behaviour by examining the complex workings of the mind, and attempt to understand processes usually considered 'normal' by the study and analysis of minds that are disturbed. The two theorists most concerned with infant development are Sigmund Freud and Erik Erikson.

Freud believed that behaviour is controlled by basic instinctual drives, sexual, life-preserving and aggressive. Life is devoted to the attempt to satisfy these drives, and it is to this end that the three structures of the psyche, the id, the ego and the superego, are developed. Conflict between these facets of the personality leads to *anxiety*, which can only be resolved if the cause of the anxiety is recognised. If the cause is not recognised, the person will fall back on defence mechanisms to reduce the stress; these mechanisms Freud believed to be 'unconscious'. Freud describes child development in terms of *psychosexual* changes; this reflects the maturational theory described above, as the transition from one stage to another was thought to be dependent on neurological development (Freud, 1965).

Erikson placed more emphasis on the 'conscious' part of the psyche, the ego, rather than on unconscious drives; his proposed stages of development are referred to as *psychosocial*. The process of development of identity is dependent on the child's interaction with the *environment and the people in it*, and is characterised by certain tasks and activities; this process continues throughout life (Erikson, 1963).

These theories on development, though different in concept, are not mutually incompatible, and seen as a whole may well give an idea of how the personality comes into being. In particular, both Freud and Erikson see the child's reaction to the caregiver as being fundamentally important in his ability to adapt to his environment later in life.

Cognitive development

There are three processes in cognitive development that seemed to D.W. Winnicott to begin very early. First, there is the process of *integration*, which is helped by all the cherishing aspects of infant care such as rocking, stroking and feeding. At this stage the baby is not aware of individuality – the ego has not yet begun to appear. Next there is *personalisation*, the gradual feeling of a person, an 'I', within the body; this feeling is partly instinctive, but will slowly become realised through 'good enough' caregiving. Lastly there is *realisation*, the beginnings of an appreciation of time, space and reality. It is through the action of the environment on the infant that he passes through the stages of absolute dependence, relative dependence and, at length, to independence (Winnicott, 1965).

Kaye (1982) sees infancy as an apprenticeship, but that it is the parents, or caregivers, who instruct and mould the being 'which must be transformed into a person'. The newborn baby is thus an organism whose mind and self will develop later in the first year; adults see the baby only as an extension of themselves, and it is their insistence on a comprehending partnership (non-existent at this time) that eventually stimulates growth and behaviour. For instance, a baby frowns with wind; the mother reads this as bad temper, as it is the sort of grimace she would make if she was angry, and she reacts to the baby by scolding him. If this reaction is repeated often enough, the baby will eventually associate the grimace with bad temper, because that is the message he is receiving. The baby therefore is conditioned by his mother into an emotional response, a process known as *classical conditioning*.

Piaget, on the other hand, did not believe that the child is shaped by the environment. His theory was that the child is the instigator of the process by actively seeking to learn from his involvement with all that is felt and seen (Piaget, 1970). The newborn baby struggles to make sense of a puzzling environment, and in so doing organises his actions. He learns to adjust physically to the maternal shape, stout or slender, and whereas at first he sucks avidly at anything that touches his mouth, eventually he will automatically turn towards the breast in search of the nipple. This is the process of *adaptation*. The baby begins to adapt to reality; at first he dreams of a nipple and one is offered – thus his fantasy is realised; after a short time the dream nipple takes form in his consciousness as an agreeable fact.

Human adults are able to 'cut out' unwanted repetitive stimuli in order to be more receptive to what is new and strange – those whose working lives are spent with the sound of clicking monitors will cease to notice this background noise and will only respond when an alarm rings, or when the machine ceases to function. They have become habituated to the sound. Newborn babies are capable of learning through *habituation*, and after a while will cease to respond with the startle reflex to repeated loud sounds. Indeed, the healthy newborn baby can, as shall be seen later, remove himself from recognised but unwanted stimuli by passing from one sleeping state to another.

All these theories and ideas are centred on one assumption – that the child develops and grows in relationship with the environment. Theorists are divided as to whether the process begins from inside-out (the baby's individual reaction to the environment) or outside-in (the impingement of the outside world on the baby). All agree, however, that the quality of this environment is of paramount importance to the infant's future well-being; for it is at this moment, when the child wakes from sleep and begins to become a person, that he is in a precarious position. Winnicott (1965) compares him to Humpty Dumpty; he has managed to climb onto the wall, but he is only too vulnerable to assault – and once off the wall, all the King's horses and all the King's men cannot put together the pieces.

Emotional development

In the newborn infant emotions are associated with bodily needs, and it is those emotions most necessary to the infant's physical well-being that develop first. How and when the development of each emotion occurs, and how this relates to the infant's cognitive ability, is the subject of different hypotheses.

The *differentiation hypothesis* holds that at the beginning there are no specific feelings, but only a generalised sensation of excitement or distress; all the other separate emotions of human experience derive from this state by a process of differentiation. This means that as the baby's personality develops, he begins to distinguish different features of his environment, and becomes capable of reacting to them with the appropriate emotion.

Sroufe (1979) saw the emotions developing in three different directions, becoming more distinct from each other with time; 'early obligatory attention' he saw differentiating into wariness, then fear; vague distress later becomes transformed into feelings of rage, anger, angry mood and defiance; and the endogenous smile of the newborn is the precursor of pleasure, laughter, joy, elation, pride and love.

The *discrete systems hypothesis* holds that each emotion develops as a separate (discrete) system, and becomes a part of the overall emotional system, all interacting with each other. Those most necessary for survival emerge first; the cry of distress, for instance, will call attention to a physical need and ensure the proximity of the caregiver. Fear, on the other hand, is not only considered as contributing little to adaptiveness in early infancy, but is also potentially dangerous, emerging only when the child begins to understand, control and needs to protect himself

(Sroufe, 1979). The effect of too premature an introduction to fear will be discussed in the next chapter.

Izard and Buechler (1979) found that expressions of emotion begin to appear at the following ages:

- At birth — interest, endogenous smile, startle, distress, disgust
- $1\frac{1}{2}$–3 months — social smile
- 2–3 months — surprise
- 3–5 months — rage and anger
- 5–9 months — fear

According to Izard and Buechler, fear, distress and anger will begin to wane or become better regulated: as the baby becomes aware of the objects and people that represent his environment; as his memory begins to develop; and as he begins to have a concept of time and space. Conception of time will lead him to understand that separation from his caregiver is only temporary – she is not here now, but will come back soon. The regulation of these stress emotions is seen by Izard and Buechler as a function of the emotion system, and a gain to the developing personality.

There are four factors that have most influence on the development of the emotion system:

- social class and environment
- dimensions of temperament
- attentional, perceptual and cognitive processes
- quality of caregiving.

All these factors will determine the way the baby and his caregiver interact with each other; that is to say, the *synchrony* between the two. This is essential to the well-being, indeed to the survival of the individual; many books have been written on the importance of synchrony between mother and child – literally, their ability to 'keep in time' with one another. It is likely that the *quality* of care given by the caregiver, and the way this is adapted to the needs of the individual baby, will have a more beneficial effect than the *quantity* of the caregiver's responses.

Emotion has a profound effect on learning, and is also associated with memory; 'the stronger the emotion the more firmly fixed the knowledge will be' (Nathan, 1988); experience of fear will remain fixed in the memory, perhaps for a lifetime.

Memory

Knowledge, experience and feelings are stored in the form of memories. Memory is not just one process but a host of different complex systems used for different purposes. The ability of environmental failure to obstruct normal emotional and cognitive development is dependent on the functions of memory; so how much (or how little) are babies able to remember, and what form will such memory take?

Functions of memory

Genetic memory is the hypothesised 'memory' for biological events occurring during the course of the evolution of the species. An example of this is the 'Moro' reflex, thought to be inherited from an instinctive ape-like grab at the mother's fur to prevent oneself from falling (Amiel-Tison & Grenier, 1986).

The *sensory information store* is a memory that lasts a very short time. After a stimulus (for instance, a heel prick) has been withdrawn, a sensory representation of the stimulus remains suspended in the mind for one or two seconds (the baby withdraws his foot away from the stimulus), and then, apparently, is lost from the store by a process of decay (the baby returns his foot to the original site of danger).

Sometimes the sensory information is passed into the *short-term memory*. This is a store of information that has received minimal processing; more than about seven items cannot be processed at a time. Once the rehearsal of the material has been interrupted it has a half-life of no more than fifteen seconds, after which it disappears (Reber, 1985).

Long-term memory is a store of information that has been coded and put away, perhaps to be recalled later as *reproductive memory*. This is reproduced or represented as something resembling the original – but it is *not* the original; *perception* draws on the coded information and reconstructs an image of what is probably there, rather than making an exact copy. Past experience, in other words, and the emotions aroused, may alter the way an object or stimulus is perceived and affect the way it is represented in the memory (Kaye, 1982).

Certain experiences can be relived, rather than recalled. Thus, for example, a certain piece of music might fill one with sadness, without one being able to recall its connection with the death of someone loved or lost in infancy. 'Music, when soft voices die, vibrates in the memory', says Shelley; the loved one has gone beyond recall, but music and sadness remain linked together. The reliving of experience has particular significance for the newborn infant, as the conclusion is that: 'the brain functions as a high-fidelity recorder, putting on tape, as it were, every experience from the time of birth, possibly even before birth' (Harris, 1973).

Memory and the CNS

Layering of the memory processes probably begins in the womb and will continue to mature at the same time as the infant's cognitive and evaluative systems (Wachter-Shikora, 1981). Memory is stored in the areas of the cortex concerned with sensory information about such things as visual patterns, location and movement (Squire, 1986). Long-term memory requires the functional ability of the limbic system and diencephalon which are already well developed in the newborn infant (Anand & Hickey, 1987). Data has shown that long-term memory in the newborn baby can exceed 24 hours, and that the infant is capable of recognising information and relating it to existing knowledge and sensory experience (Papoušek & Papoušek, 1983; Mussen *et al.*, 1984). The infant may be able to relate previous experiences to previous happenings as early as two months of age, and will be attracted by objects that fit into a familiar pattern (Minde & Minde, 1986).

Unconscious memory

Birth trauma can have a profound effect later in life, as discussed in Chapter 2. Adults can relive the pain of circumcision, and graphically describe the event. A child reacts violently to every association that reminds him of horrific pain inflicted in infancy (Chamberlain, 1989); but although memory is present and functioning at an unconscious level at a very early age, it cannot always be put into words or recollected in verbal form: 'These were my thoughts; I kept them to myself, for at that age I had not learnt to speak', says Hilarion in the Gilbert and Sullivan opera *Princess Ida*. He kept them to himself in the storage space for 'unnamed' images which is the unconscious.

But the unconscious is not the dead storage space of a basement full of dusty old books; it is more like storing a family of rabbits: 'these rabbits, fed by the feelings of the moment, breed and grow more powerful and would soon overrun the mind completely if they were not released' (Berne, 1986). Unfortunately, tensions cannot be released all in one go, but must be drained off regularly over a lifetime, and just releasing a few rabbits at a time is not going to prevent more rabbits from arriving by the dozen. If this storage space of feelings is packed with negative images due to unconscious memories of unremitting aggression, it is not surprising if later on the released rabbits have turned into wolves.

Chapter 2
Awakening to Suffering

The trauma of being born

There are dozens of articles on the pains of labour suffered by the mother, and how they may be alleviated. Few refer to the travail of the baby, yet this passage between the harmony that is experienced in the womb and the discordance of a world that demands to be noticed is a trauma at least as shocking for the baby as the mother. The narcissistic newborn baby who exists within himself, must now shift his attention to what is without. Within, all was warmth and dimness and muffled sound; without, nothing but cold and light and noise.

There is no way for a baby to avoid the trauma of the birth experience, and now he faces a period of great change. He no longer floats in substances that gently stroke the skin, but is deposited naked and raw on his mother's bosom, or is bundled away into a cot, where his limbs weigh heavily upon him; now that he is subjected for the first time to the laws of gravity, he must feel as strange as a space traveller returned to earth.

The baby has many different ways of reacting to this change; sometimes he cries, sometimes he looks about him in wondering silence, sometimes he searches blindly to suck, sometimes he collapses into a state of white and breathless shock from which he will recover only with difficulty. Small wonder that this period is thought by many psychiatrists to have a life-long effect on the individual.

Many people unconsciously remember the trauma of their own birth, and use vivid imagery to express their feelings and memories: 'a bridge from one mode of existence to another', 'a chiasma', 'a hiatus', 'a kind of blackout closely resembling death', are some of the phrases used (Greenacre, 1953). Greenacre believed that the special traumatic experiences of the passage through the birth canal, together with the contrast between the total dependence of existence in the womb and the quasi-dependence of life 'outside', might, combined with genetic elements, be factors contributing to a 'predisposition to anxiety'. The idea that birth experiences seem to organise an individual's anxiety pattern was also believed by Freud. But birth is an experience common to all, and most babies weather the storm.

Environmental failure and ego development

The effects of early excessive painful experience may present later in life as an anxious attitude itself – 'the sense that something unpleasant or positively painful will happen' (Greenacre, 1953). But a baby that never experiences discomfort and is always completely satisfied will lose a certain healthy aggression and stimulation, and become restless. Since there is no such thing as a 'perfect mother', the care of an infant will always be deficient to some degree, and the resultant anxiety felt by the baby was considered normal by Winnicott (1975). This failure to meet all the baby's needs is known as the graduated failure, and it will in time enable the baby to discriminate between the environment 'outside' as opposed to the self 'inside' – but this progression must be gradual; the developing psyche is not yet sufficiently strong to resist constant bombardment of influences from the outside world. If the reaction required from the baby is beyond his capabilities, it may lead to an extreme sense of insecurity and loss of identity: 'a congenital ... hopelessness in respect of the attainment of a personal life' (Winnicott, 1975); the response will be withdrawal and regression.

The same argument was presented by the psychoanalyst Michael Balint in his book *The Basic Fault* (1968); 'fault' was the word used by many of his patients to describe a feeling that for almost all of their lives there had been something missing within them that must be put right. The origin of this fault Balint could trace back to a considerable discrepancy in the early formative years of the individual between his physical and emotional needs and the care and attention he received at this time; a discrepancy which leaves a sense of deficiency persisting into adult life. The cause of this discrepancy may be congenital, or failure of the environment 'such as care that is insufficient, deficient, haphazard, over-anxious, over-protective, harsh, rigid, grossly inconsistent, incorrectly timed, over-stimulating, or merely un-understanding or indifferent ... I put the emphasis on the lack of "fit" between the child and the people who represent his environment' (Balint, 1968).

Helplessness, fear, depression, persecution

Human infants are more helpless at birth than any other species, and, since they are unable to take care of themselves, have to submit to whatever treatment they receive. Most will gradually develop some form of mastery over their surroundings, as with time the response of their caregivers to their demands teaches them the correlation between cause and effect. But 'responsive mothering is fundamental to the learning of mastery. Absence of mothering, stimulus deprivation and non-responsive mothering all contribute to the learning of uncontrollability' (Seligmann, 1975). When the newborn baby cries, mother is expected to appear with food, clean nappies and cuddles. An infant deprived of this sort of satisfaction is an infant deprived of mastery. The overdisciplined NU, where food, clean nappies and cuddles arrive at the stroke of the clock and not because the baby has asked for them, offer him no conception of his own power as a controller of events.

At the other extreme, if infants subjected to pain find that their reactions evoke no response but only fall into a vacuum, the result will be the impotent rage of the entirely helpless: '*Helplessness* in an infant has the same consequences as in an adult: lack of response initiation, difficulty in seeing that responding works, anxiety and depression' (Seligmann, 1975). If this goes on for long the baby will cease to respond at all; not only this, but he will learn that responding does not matter. This is disastrous for an infant; it means that if protest and resistance to a painful object do not lead to escape, protest becomes meaningless. If he cannot control trauma by being afraid and acting on his fear, then *fear* will be replaced by *depression*. Fear is useful in that it forces us to defend ourselves or try to escape. If the escape mechanism fails to work, then fear becomes irrelevant: 'it is worse than useless since it costs the subject great energy in a hopeless situation. Depression then ensues' (Seligmann, 1975). And energy is something the fragile newborn infant cannot afford to waste.

In some cases, early prolonged traumatic experience can be recalled later as *persecution*; the result of this may be that the infant needs and welcomes persecution, as only then does he have a sense of reality: 'But this represents a false mode of development, since the infant needs continued persecution' (Winnicott, 1975). In 1983 Herzog described 'An Intensive Care Syndrome': a condition of 'needing pain' observed in some small children who had undergone prolonged traumatic experiences in infancy. The children would do anything they could to provoke violence against themselves.

We can safely assume, then, that unrelenting pressure from the world on the developing consciousness of the newborn baby, before he is ready to assimilate it, may have harmful consequences later. We have seen that pain can be remembered; when birth trauma is significant every detail of impingement and reaction is etched on the memory to be relived with other painful experiences later in life: 'Among features of the true birth memory is the feeling of being in the grip of something external, so that one is helpless ... the intolerable nature of experiencing something without any knowledge whatever of when it will end' (Winnicott, 1975). If this is the effect of birth trauma – a transitory experience – what can be etched on the memory of the infant subjected to the prolonged and relentless trauma of intensive care, with its attendant invasions of the person? Humpty Dumpty's shell is fragile, it is dangerous to knock him off the wall; he needs to be supported so that he can sit there in safety, absorbing all he sees.

The preterm infant

The foetus exists as an extension of the mother and is entirely dependent on her for nourishment, protection and well-being. If something occurs to impair this relationship the foetus will no longer be able to thrive and the function of the uterus will become inhibiting rather than cherishing. That the foetus can be physiologically affected by adverse conditions during pregnancy is well known; such factors as pre-eclamptic toxaemia, maternal infection, malnutrition, alcohol and drug abuse may harm the growing infant irrecoverably. But it has been shown that psychological stress in the mother may also have an adverse effect on her unborn child. 'Life-events' stress experienced in early pregnancy can predispose the infant to physical abnormalities at birth, and behavioural problems later on; and there may well be a connection in later pregnancy between life-events stress and stillbirth and neonatal death (Connolly & Cullen, 1983).

When the womb ceases to be undemanding and neutral, the foetus will have more chance of survival in the exterior world, but the so-called 'paradise' of the post-natal state is not available to the preterm infant in the NU. The preterm infant has no mastery over his surroundings, since without the aid of technology he would be unable to survive. He is at the mercy of sensations against which he is incapable of defending himself, and inappropriate experience of the world outside the womb will not only inhibit ego development, but also have a damaging effect on the rapidly developing foetal brain (see Chapter 3). He has all the potential, if he can be kept alive long enough, to eventually grow into a 'normal' baby. But in the meantime he lives a manufactured life, kept breathing by mechanical means, fed artificially, and lying solitary in a perspex box constantly observed from outside. If we accept that the preterm infant is not an inadequate or deficient term infant but a 'well-equipped, competently adapted organism appropriately functioning at his stage and his environment' (Als, 1986), we can readily understand that the extra-uterine environment in which he now finds himself is unsuitable, even bizarre, and he will be incapable of reacting in an organised way. Caregivers need to supply the 'responsive mothering' which will offer the immature infant support until such time as he can begin to 'master his surroundings'.

Long-term effects of environmental failure

In hospital

NICUs have been described as sensorily depriving, excessively stimulating, or providing dissociated patterns of stimulation (Gottfried *et al.*, 1984). Babies have shown their individuality by reacting to this intrusive environment in different ways; some infants appear active and confident; more sensitive babies create a defensive shell in order to survive (Fig. 2.1) (Huteau, 1988; Sparshott, 1991b). This can be entirely useful if it is of short duration; in the course of development the baby will 'peck his way out'. However, prolonged retreat behind this protective shell can become pathological, and the baby will behave like Shakespeare's snail 'whose horns being hit, Shrinks backwards in his shelly cave with pain, And there all smother'd up, in shade doth sit, Long after fearing to creep forth again'. That a supportive environment supplied to babies in hospital can have a beneficial effect was demonstrated by Heidelise Als (1986). She established that attention to an individual infant's cues, and a consequent adaptation of caregiving behaviour and control of input from the environment, would improve medical and developmental outcome, and increase his chances of a good relationship with his parents: 'the highly volatile, poorly regulated, hypersensitive and overactive baby was expected to place a very different demand on his caregiving parents than the well-regulated baby at the same weight and sucking ability'.

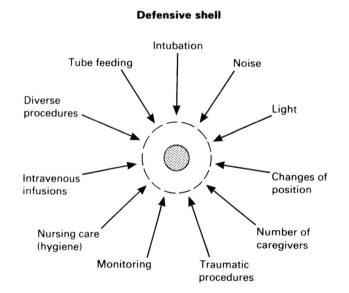

Fig. 2.1. Preterm infant stress factors. (Adapted from Sparshott, 1991c.)

Schraeder (1986) also showed that a good 'holding' environment can do much to repair the adverse effects of the early experiences of the very light birth weight (VLBW) infant. Development may in fact be more sensitive to a subsequently supportive environment than to perinatal trauma, and as the child grows older so the influence of the 'good' environment will increase and the impact of the original 'bad' environment will decrease. Two reasons were given for this: the first was the self-regulatory abilities of the child; preterm babies may be thrown off course, but once an appropriate environment is established for them they will be brought back onto the right trajectory. The other reason given was that the child would grow *in the context* of this good environment – like a delicate seedling kept in the dark who is at last exposed to sun and warmth.

At home

The importance of a supportive home environment for babies who have been hospitalised at birth is underlined in many studies of developmental progress: 'the effect of low birth weight is seen to be most marked in children who have the added disadvantages of an adverse home background and a poor genetic endowment' (Drillien, 1964); behavioural and emotional problems have led to such children being described as over-anxious, shy and passive, or aggressive. A study investigating the development of full term infants who required intensive care at birth found that at one year they were performing significantly less well than a control group in almost all areas. Three factors appeared to play an important role: the length of the infant's stay in hospital, the severity of the illness, and the mother's psychiatric state; the association between the mother's state and the infant's development seems to indicate that a depressed mother interacts less with her baby in the early months, possibly due to the fact that the 'sick' infant is unresponsive and will not 'play' (Ludman *et al.*, 1989).

Other studies have demonstrated problems in temperament and behaviour in very preterm infants, and those who have been subjected to intensive care (Field *et al.*, 1978; Washington *et al.*, 1986). Yet Oberklaid *et al.* (1991) found little difference in behaviour and temperament between preterm and term infants at six years of age; indeed, as young toddlers the preterm infants seemed more likely to be 'easy' and less likely to be 'difficult'. More than half the preterm infants examined during this study, however, were over 33 weeks gestational age, and the researchers conceded the VLBW infants who suffer significant perinatal stress and medical complications and whose home environment is not supportive are more likely to have problems of temperament later on.

The consensus of opinion seems to be that the high risk infant, who has managed to survive the traumas of intensive care, tends to catch up gradually, so that by the time he goes to school there are relatively few deficits – but this will depend on the environment with which he is provided, both in hospital and at home. If he can be maintained in a state of relative well-being – and is not subjected to repeated traumatic experiences without relief – the preterm infant with a stable family background may well start off to school 'with shining morning face' like any other child.

Chapter 3
Pain, Distress and Nervous System Development

The nervous system is described as 'the mechanism whereby the individual is enabled to react to his environment, and whereby the various activities of the body are correlated and controlled' (Nathan, 1988). It is important for caregivers to understand the stages at which the central and autonomic nervous systems develop in the foetus, otherwise we will be unable to supply a suitable environment for the preterm infant's individual needs. We must also be aware of the potential hazards to these systems, and their probable consequences. And, above all, we must recognise to what extent the developing CNS is sensitive to pain; although in this context it has been suggested that nociceptive activity would be a better term to use, since the word 'pain' has now come to include such variables as social background, emotional and psychological response, previous experience and memory (Anand & Hickey, 1987; Anand, 1993).

The central nervous system

Environmental failure and CNS development

It has been suggested by many specialists that neurological development can be influenced by sensory input from the environment; stimuli encountered by the eyes, for example, may affect the growth of the visual system. This concerns the biochemical manifestation of memory called the *engram*: a biochemical change brought about by external stimulation, leading to a permanent alteration of neural tissue that represents what has been learned (Reber, 1985). Sensory experiences that influence neurological development begin during the later stages of foetal development. Instead of the womb, however, the preterm infant at this sensitive moment of neurological growth is subjected to stimuli from the NICU; not only the cognitive and emotional development, but also the biological strata of such development, the structure and functions of the CNS, may be influenced by the quality of input from the environment.

Experience of pain in infancy therefore may well prove to be the most critical determinant of future responses to pain.

That transitory pain leaves only short-term imprint on the memory is suggested by the fact that the hurt baby, after drawing his limb away, will immediately return it to the site of the injury. But many of the systems of the brain responsible for memory are active at birth, as we have seen in Chapter 1; it is simply that the baby has yet to learn the hard lesson of 'cause and effect'. *Cognitive* development begins at birth, maybe before – the experience of pain has to be assimilated along with other experiences of life. We also need to know to what extent the baby is *neurologically* capable of pain experience.

The following are some milestones in the development of the foetal central and autonomic nervous systems as they concern the pain pathway, followed by reference to some of the dangers inherent in inappropriate stimulation (Als, 1986; Anand & Hickey, 1987; White-Traut *et al.*, 1994).

The neurons

The density of the nociceptive nerve endings in the skin is comparable with, if not greater than, that in the skin of an adult. Cutaneous receptors begin to appear in the area of the mouth in the 7th week' g.a., then spread to the palms of the hands and the soles of the feet by the 11th week, and to the trunk and proximal parts of the limbs by the 15th week. By 20 weeks' g.a., nerve endings have spread to all cutaneous and mucous surfaces.

The spinal cord

The spread of cutaneous receptors is preceded by the development of synapses between sensory fibres and interneurons in the dorsal horn of the spinal cord, which already begins to appear during the 6th week g.a. The development of various types of cells together with their laminar arrangement, synaptic interconnections and specific neurotransmitter vesicles begins before 13 to 14 weeks' g.a., and by 30 weeks is completed (Anand & Hickey, 1987).

Myelination

One of the arguments in favour of lack of pain perception in the newborn and preterm infant has been the supposed lack of myelination of the nerve fibres; but nociceptive impulses are carried through the thinly myelinated A delta and C unmyelinated fibres which, though they transmit slowly, have shorter distances to travel in the newborn baby. In any case, it is now known that myelination throughout the CNS is completed during the 2nd and 3rd trimester. Myelination of nociceptors in the spinal cord is completed between 8 and 12 weeks' g.a. By 30 weeks, pathways to the brain stem and thalamus concerned with pain are completely myelinated.

Myelination can, however, be interrupted or disturbed by severe dehydration and malnutrition, and by periventricular leukomalacia (PVL), a necrotic lesion in the area of and adjacent to the external angles of the lateral ventricles of the brain (Als, 1986; Anand & Hickey, 1987; Van der Bor *et al.*, 1989). Van der Bor *et al.* used magnetic resonance imaging to show that PVL is associated with delayed brain development, *particularly* delayed myelination.

The brain

The midbrain and limbic system

Cells in the cerebral cortex originate in germinal layers lining the ventricular system. While this germinal layer is producing brain cells it contains many blood vessels. Between 8 and 26 weeks, afferent nerve cells produce axons which travel towards the cortex before midgestation; they then 'wait' for the neurons in the cortex to mature, finally establishing synaptic connections between 20 and 24 weeks' g.a. Each new cell migrates through the thickness of the cortex to its specific place on the surface. These cells then develop dendrites which link up with other cells in order to transmit impulses (Anand & Hickey, 1987; Bellig, 1989; White-Traut *et al.*, 1994).

At 26 to 28 weeks' g.a. the germinal matrix is still full of tiny blood vessels which supply oxygen to produce the cells of the cortex. Since many of these cells have already migrated, the tissue is lax, unsupported, and thus susceptible to haemorrhage. A sharp increase in blood pressure inside the head is apt to rupture these vessels and lead to cerebral haemorrhage of varying degrees of severity (Als, 1986). Since most of the sensory pathways synapse in the thalamus, this period is of vital importance to the growing foetus; damage or delay at this stage is irreparable.

The cerebral cortex

Compared with an adult brain which is only 2% of body weight, the brain of a newborn baby is large, comprising 12% of the infant's total body weight. It begins to mature from the centre, development progressing from the medulla oblongata and the brain stem outwards to the cortex; conditioned reflexes which involve the brain stem therefore appear before birth, unconditioned reflexes coming later as the cortex develops. This development begins in the foetus at 8 weeks' g.a.; by 20 weeks the cortex has a full complement of 10^9 neurons, and new cells are probably formed up to 40 weeks. Up to 5 years of age, synapses continue to be established rapidly, probably continuing at a slower pace until 18 years (Anand & Hickey, 1987).

At 15 weeks' g.a. the cerebral hemispheres are smooth, but by 40 weeks the convolutions of sulci and gyri have multiplied to such an extent that the surface of the cortex covers twice the visible area (Crawford, 1994). More and more sulci appear as cells become larger and more elaborately connected. The right side of the brain organises two weeks before the left – assymetry is normal between sides (Als, 1986). Specialisations associated with the two sides of the cerebral hemispheres are now generally considered to come about slowly and may be associated with sex differences. Complex functions associated with the frontal lobes, such as problem solving, also develop slowly (Bee, 1985).

The functional maturity of the cortex can be seen by studying electroencephalogramic patterns, cerebral metabolism and the behaviour of newborn infants. Intermittent bursts are first seen on electroencephalogram at 20 weeks' g.a.; by 30 weeks distinction can be made by this means between sleeping and waking, although the pattern remains immature. Measurements of cerebral glucose utilisation have shown maximal metabolic activity in the sensory areas of the brain (sensory-motor cortex, thalamus, midbrain and brain stem). Besides this, the reactions of preterm and full term infants to such stimuli as light and sound show the functional ability of the cortex (Anand & Hickey, 1987).

After 32 to 34 weeks' g.a., the richest blood supply is found in the mid zone of the cortex; changes in blood pressure can lead to multiple small infarcts in the periventricular areas. Intracerebellar haemorrhage can also be caused by obstruction of blood vessels through external compression, such as constriction by oxygen mask, posterior pressure on the head through lying in an unsupported supine position, or the fixing of an endotracheal tube (Als, 1986; Emery, 1996).

Maturation of the white matter of the brain can also be inhibited by PVL, which is frequently associated with cerebral palsy; one of the risk factors for this condition is frequent episodes of bradycardia and apnoea, resulting in hyperfusion and ischaemia (Pape & Wigglesworth, 1979; Monset-Couchard *et al.*, 1988; Pidcock *et al.*, 1990).

Chemical neurotransmitters

Substance P and its receptors begin to appear in the dorsal root ganglia and the dorsal horns of the spinal cord at 12 to 16 weeks' g.a. Substance

P fibres and cells have also been found in the limbic and midbrain areas and in the cerebral cortex of foetuses early in their development. Research has shown that a higher density of substance P and its receptors is found in the newborn than in adults, though the significance of this is not known (Anand & Hickey, 1987).

Stress in newborn infants undergoing surgery and following traumatic procedures can be indicated by hormonal and metabolic changes; catecholamine release can be a strong indication of stress (Anand, 1986; 1993). Chemical pain regulators such as the endogenous opioids have been found at birth in infants subjected to stress, sometimes in quantities three to five times greater than in adults. Beta endorphin and beta litrophin levels have been recorded at exceptionally high levels in infants delivered by Caesarian section, breech presentation or vacuum extraction, and also in infants suffering from birth asphyxia, hypoxia, apnoea of prematurity and infection. This high level may be due to the stress of illness, the experience of pain and discomfort, or the invasive procedures used in treatment. The raised levels of endogenous opioids decrease rapidly over a period of 24 hours, and at the end of 5 days have often reached adult levels (Anand & Hickey, 1987).

Neurotransmitters are often only released if up to four or five different regulatory systems occur in a specific order. The density and sensitivity of receptors for certain neurotransmitters vary with different regions of the brain and are influenced by experience, since brain and sensory organs depend upon each other for the normal development of structure and function (Als, 1986).

Development of sensory function

The following summarises briefly the order in appearance of sensory function (White-Traut *et al.*, 1994):

(1) Cutaneous (tactile) function commences during the first 2 months' gestation; by 10 to 12 weeks' g.a. there is a differentiation of response (Gottlieb, 1971).
(2) Taste buds are formed at 11 weeks' g.a., and are functioning by 12 weeks' g.a. (Bradley & Stern, 1967).
(3) Olfactory function appears by 3rd trimester (Sarnat, 1978).
(4) Auditory system is fully functional by 25 to 27 weeks' g.a. (Rubel, 1985).
(5) Vision achieves functional status only approaching the last trimester; even then colour vision is poorly developed (Munsinger, 1970). Response to light has been recorded at 22 weeks' g.a. (Engel, 1964).

It is therefore evident that the baby has all the somatic sensory equipment necessary for the perception of painful stimuli, as well as the neurological and chemical systems involved, at birth or even before.

Overstimulation by light and sound can be harmful to the immature infant, as shown in Chapter 8, but appropriate stimulation of sensory function is beneficial. In the NU most attention is paid to stimulation of the auditory and visual capabilities of the infant. If, as shown above, touch, taste and smell are the first sensory functions to appear, it would seem that stimulation of these sensations would be valuable, particularly as, for the fragile infant, most tactile experience comes in the form of medical and nursing procedures, and is therefore likely to be aggressive. Positive results have been seen from taste, smell and tactile stimulation during episodes of apnoea (Garcia & White-Traut, 1993), and tactile and kinesthetic stimulation has also been shown to have a beneficial effect on sympathetic and adrenocortical function in preterm infants (Kuhn *et al*, 1991).

Consequences of developmental impairment

Modern technology has improved the survival rates of preterm infants; they are also becoming viable at an increasingly early age. However, follow up indicates that the preterm infant, especially if less than 32 weeks' g.a., may later show evidence of neuromotor abnormalities, learning disabilities and behaviour problems, which have been identified even when intraventricular haemorrhage and bronchopulmonary dysplasia (BPD) do not appear to be present (Als *et al.*, 1986). Where there is no damage to the brain, developmental impairment would therefore appear to occur because the foetal nervous system is not adapted for extrauterine life, suggesting that the cellular growth of the brain is also influenced by the environment through the senses: touch, taste, smell, sound and sight. Studies of animal brains show that the sensitive period of brain development between 26 and 40 weeks' g.a. requires a finely tuned and balanced support from the environment. Normally this period is spent in the uterus, but, as we saw in the previous chapter, even this may not be safe if the infant is undernourished or affected by maternal stress. Malnutrition in early pregnancy is likely to lead to decreased cell number and decreased brain size; later, malnutrition may hinder myelinisation, denditric arborisation and nerve cell transmission (Bellig, 1989); alterations in cerebral functioning could lead to changes in the enzyme composition of the brain (McIlwain, 1970).

The *pattern* of brain development, in other words, may be modified by early experience. Development may be distorted if the generation of nervous system pathways is inhibited or suppressed due to overactivation of pathways already functioning. These suppressions appear to be mediated by endorphin mechanisms (chemical transmitters) associated with the cortical areas of the frontal cortex; areas associated with attention, learning and behaviour. The presence of neuro-transmitters seems to be dependent on the correct sequential development and functioning of these areas of the cortex. That is, the areas of the brain must develop at a specific rate and in a specific order if one area is not to overdevelop at the expense of another. Since all the different parts of the brain are interdependent, damage in one area may be seen later to have had a 'rippling effect' on the other areas; failure to function correctly in one system will always be reflected in the others. Inappropriate experience may lead to overstimulation of one area, with the consequent deprivation of another (Als, 1986). If it is provided with the proper support and appropriate stimulation, however, the immature brain compensates and will continue to develop and progress normally.

Synactive organisation of behavioural development

Once the shock of being born has passed, the preterm infant will try to re-establish the level of developmental activity arrived at before 'shut down'. The capacity of the preterm infant for self-regulation is limited, however; he will therefore require appropriate support and stimulation from caregivers to assist and sustain balanced CNS development. This will entail the balancing of the various interacting subsystems which make up the whole individual system of behaviour. Als (1986) designed a 'model of the synactive organization of behavioural development' to aid caregivers in 'the protection and support of the immature yet rapidly differentiating brain in our NICU environments'. This shows how that brain's functional integrity can be reflected in the infant's behaviour. During synactive development, *five subsystems of functioning* are continuously interacting. Confronted by pressures from the environment, each baby shows his individuality by displaying his ability to integrate each subsystem with the others. These subsystems are:

- the autonomic and physiological system
- the motor system
- the state system
- the attentional-interactive system
- the self-regulatory system (strategies employed by the infant as he adjusts to his surroundings).

Before such integration takes place, however, the infant must have developed adequate internal stability and cohesion; as a general rule preterm infants should be able to accommodate social interaction by 33 weeks' g.a., but of course each baby needs to be assessed on an individual basis. Close observation of behaviour and monitoring of physiological signs will be necessary to protect the fragile infant from potentially harmful stimulation, particularly when brain damage is present (White-Traut *et al.*, 1993).

It is apparent, then, that the brain of the preterm infant, rather than being too immature to register and process sensory information, is in fact hypersensitive. Adequate nutrition, attention to ante-natal care, relief of stress during pregnancy, and maintenance of an appropriate environment for the preterm infant, will all help to minimise the many obstacles threatening the correct sequential development of the burgeoning CNS. The subsystems of functioning as expressed by infant behaviour can be used to enable caregivers to adapt the environment of the NU to the needs of each individual baby, in ways which will be discussed in Chapter 4.

Chapter 4
Infant Behaviour

'I choose to wonder how babies manage to pass the time ... well, partly they sleep/And mostly they weep/And the rest of the time they relax/On their backs', said the poet Ogden Nash. Of course he was joking, but this is in fact a very good description of the 'states of consciousness' in which babies pass their first few months of life. Since the baby's reception of the world will depend on his ongoing state, we need to be able to identify these states in order to respond appropriately to each baby's individual needs.

States of consciousness

The newborn infant shows behaviour that may be described as *endogenous*; that is to say, behaviour that seems to have its origin within the baby himself, and does not appear to be influenced by outside events. For example, many movements made by the baby at this time are diffuse and apparently meaningless, suggesting an isolation from, or at least an incomprehension of, the world about him (Minde & Minde, 1986). These internal activities, described as states of consciousness or sleep/wake states were used as a basis for the Neonatal Behavioral Assessment Scale (NBAS) of Brazelton & Nugent (1995) (Table 4.1 and Fig. 4.1).

The passage through the states of consciousness represents the daily life of the baby's internal world. The states of consciousness occur in a cycle which, in a newborn infant, is repeated every one-and-a-half to two hours – the baby moves from deep sleep to light sleep to drowsiness to alertness to fussy wakefulness to hunger, and then once satisfied to deep sleep again; as time progresses he may link some of these states together without becoming fully awake, and it is at this point we say that he 'sleeps through the night' (Bee, 1985).

This apparently boring daily life is in fact full of activity and business. The body and brain of an infant grow rapidly during the first year, and he is learning all the time. A baby in the period of light sleep may behave much like a dog dreaming of rabbits; his eyelids flutter, and he may

Table 4.1   States of consciousness.

Sleep states

Deep sleep – with regular breathing, eyes closed, no spontaneous activity except startles or jerky movements at quite regular intervals; external stimuli produce startles with some delay; suppression of startles is rapid, and state changes are less likely than from other states. No eye movements (State 1).

Light sleep – with eyes closed; rapid eye movements (REM) can often be observed under closed lids; low activity level, with random movements and startles or startle equivalents; movements are likely to be smoother and more monitored than in State 1; responds to internal and external stimuli with startle equivalents, often with a resulting change of state. Respirations are irregular, sucking movements occur off and on (State 2). Eye opening may occur briefly at intervals.

Awake states

Drowsy – or semi-dozing; eyes may be open but dull and heavy-lidded, or closed, eyelids fluttering; activity level variable, with interspersed, mild startles from time to time; reactive to sensory stimuli, but response often delayed; state change after stimulation frequently noted. Movements are usually smooth. Dazed look when the infant is not processing information and is not 'available' (State 3).

Alert – with bright look; seems to focus invested attention on source of stimulation, such as an object to be sucked, or a visual or auditory stimulus; impinging stimuli may break through, but with some delay in response. Motor activity is at a minimum. There is a kind of glazed look which can be easily broken through in this state (State 4).

Considerable motor activity – eyes open; considerable motor activity, with thrusting movements of the extremities, and even a few spontaneous startles; reactive to external stimulation with increase in startles or motor activity, but discrete reactions difficult to distinguish because of general activity level. Brief fussy vocalisations occur in this state (State 5).

Crying – characterised by intense crying which is difficult to break through with stimulation; motor activity is high (State 6).

(From Brazelton & Nugent, 1995, courtesy of Mac Keith Press, London.)

twitch and make little sounds and grimaces. What exactly is going on at this time we have no means of knowing, but REM sleep is believed to be a time of intense stimulation of the CNS, and it seems likely that the baby is 'processing' some of the new experiences with which he is being bombarded (Bee, 1985).

Peter Wolff (1966), described by Minde and Minde as 'one of the first scientific baby watchers', linked the internal 'state' of the healthy term baby with his ability to receive stimuli from and respond to the environment. During *deep sleep*, an intense external stimulus can evoke a response (a sudden loud noise or sharp pain for example), but usually it is the baby's own 'biological clock' which will awaken him, not the movements of ordinary life around him. For this reason, parents do not really need to protect the baby during the day from the sounds of

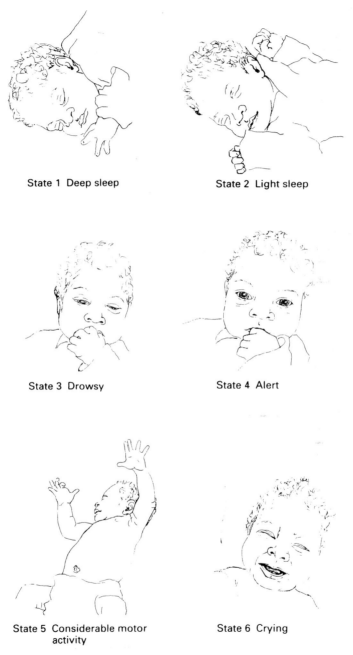

Fig. 4.1 States of consciousness. (Adapted from Brazelton & Nugent, 1995, courtesy of Mac Keith Press, London.)

children playing and dogs barking – the baby will become habituated to this and will sleep through it.

When the baby is *alert* and comfortable – nappy dry, hunger satisfied – he will begin to attend to his immediate environment. He can also be aroused from a drowsy or fussy state when distracted by something that catches his interest – but his attention span is short, and the 'alert' inactive state disappears as soon as the interesting spectacle is removed. Sooner or later, hunger or other discomforts distract the baby, and then no attempt to beguile him will draw his attention from physical needs. When the infant is *crying*, either he is defending himself against stimulation from an outside world which is too overwhelming, or he is struggling against equally overwhelming feelings of discomfort. Normally crying will conjure up food and clean nappies, and the baby will sleep again. If he is not satisfied, however, unless fatigue or some other consoling action from the caregiver intervenes, crying can progress to a state of *tantrum*; a state of yelling and exaggerated motor activity (Wolff, 1966).

Assessment of infant behaviour

Several systems have been developed to assist doctors and nurses in their assessment of newborn babies; routinely used are the Apgar and Dubowitz scores, but others evolved to assess infant behaviour include the Graham-Rosenblith Score, the Neurological and Adaptive Capacity Score (NACS), Brazelton's Neonatal Behavioral Assessment Scale (NBAS), and the Assessment of Preterm Infant Behavior (APIB).

The *Graham-Rosenblith Score* was a modification of the Graham Behavioural Test, and was designed to outline the difference in the behaviour of newborn babies in their response to individual stimuli (Rosenblith, 1961). It is interesting to note that the original score devised by Graham included a test for an infant's pain threshold (Graham *et al.*, 1956).

The *Neurological and Adaptive Capacity Score* (NACS), sometimes known as ABS after the first letters of Amiel-Tison, Barrier and Shnider, who in 1982 were principally concerned with its creation, was designed for use with full term infants; it included adaptive capacity (response and habituation to sound and light, consolability), passive and active tone, primary reflexes and general assessment (alertness, crying, motor activity). This scoring system has the advantage of being sensitive to the possible deleterious effects of drugs, as it emphasises muscle tone; also it does not require the repeated use of potentially disturbing stimuli in order to provoke a response (Amiel-Tison & Grenier, 1986).

The Neonatal Behavioral Assessment Scale (NBAS)

The NBAS, first devised by T. Berry Brazelton in 1973, is concerned with the behavioural evaluation of term babies and their interaction with their caregivers. In the NBAS the infant is seen as 'a social organism' who seems to be 'predisposed to interact with (his) caregiver from the beginning' (Brazelton & Nugent, 1995), and the test is designed to assess his ability to manage his physiological system in response to external stimulation and handling. The NBAS was designed to elicit the *optimal* response from the baby, so it is usually performed midway between feeds, when the baby is neither hungry nor sleepy, but is in the alert state. The infant's state of consciousness is an important factor; patterns of state change and state lability in response to external and internal stimuli are recorded over the course of the examination.

The advantage of the NBAS is that it emphasises interaction between infant and caregiver; official training is needed for clinical use if the responses are to be elicited in a standard manner, and training centres have been established for this purpose (Appendix 4). The NBAS can also be used to help parents understand their baby's individual needs. Demonstration of the scale to parents, together with explanation and interpretation of behaviour, has proved of value in the promotion of a positive relationship between parent and child (Brazelton & Nugent, 1995).

Methods of communication

Since speech is not available to the newborn infant, observation of behavioural reactions to stimulation must serve instead as an indication of his needs. Brazelton describes the actions taken by a newborn baby to calm and control himself as he passes from a quiet state to fussiness; he performs a hand-to-mouth movement – maybe even sucks his fist – and, as he relaxes, looks about for something to take his interest. Once alert, he is capable of periods of active attention, fixing his gaze and turning his head to follow the movement of an attractive visual stimulus, and responding to auditory stimuli by either turning towards a sound with interest, or showing dislike by jerky movements and startles, crying, or even a state of controlled inactivity resembling sleep. In this state he 'shuts out' stimuli, and protects himself by withdrawing from the proceedings: face mask-like; eyes tightly closed; body and limbs tightly held. If, during a 'shutting out' state, the baby is offered a sound he finds agreeable, such as a soft rattle or soothing human voice, he may respond by returning to an alert state, turning eyes and head towards the source of the attractive sound (Brazelton, 1961).

The individual behavioural responses of a newborn baby will also influence the feelings of the caregiver. As well as response to visual and auditory stimuli, the movements of the baby when he is cuddled – the way he moulds his body when held in the arms, and snuggles his head into the caregiver's neck when held against the shoulder – all stimulate attraction. The ability of the infant to beguile is assessed in the NBAS as *cuddliness*, a summary measure of the infant's response to being held whilst in an alert state. The infant who does not participate but lies passively 'like a sack of meal' may repel the examiner – he is 'glad to be finished'. On the other hand, the baby who moulds and relaxes disarms the examiner, and would be 'enjoyable to take home'! (Brazelton, 1984).

The NBAS has been the basis for many studies of behaviour following traumatic procedures. It was used by Marshall *et al.,* (1982) to assess changes in behaviour following circumcision effected by means of a clamp, with the baby strapped down on a circumcision board that fixed arms and legs immobile. Hardly surprisingly, it was found that 90% of infants showed changes in behaviour after this procedure, and in 33% these changes lasted for at least 22 hours. An interesting behavioural trend was observed from this study: 83% of babies who were crying at the commencement of the operation became hyperactive afterwards, whereas those who had been in a quiet alert state became less active. Was this due to differences in personality, or a response to the conflicting instincts of fight and fright?

Assessment of Preterm Infant Behaviour (APIB)

The concentration demanded by the NBAS would be likely to stress the autonomic state control of the fragile or preterm infant, whose reactions are in any case less likely to be organised than those of a well baby born at term. For this reason, the APIB was adapted from the NBAS as an instrument for assessing the behaviour of preterm infants, and was designed to highlight the capacity of the fragile infant to absorb information – this capacity being one measure of fragility and/or immaturity (Als *et al.,* 1982).

The APIB is based on the synactive theory of infant development discussed in Chapter 3. Unlike the well baby at term, a preterm, sick or disorganised baby spends most of his time in REM sleep; periods of deep sleep are rare. He may be incapable of passing from one sleeping/waking state to another in order to control levels of stimulation, and by either over-reacting to or 'turning off' the outside world he might well affect his first interactions with his parents or caregivers, and influence his future relationship with them (Als *et al.,* 1982). The fragile infant demonstrates overstimulation by certain signs of instability (withdrawal behaviour) associated with the function of the subsystems; likewise he will respond with signs of stability (approach behaviour) when in a state of well-being; these are summarised in Table 4.2.

The APIB can be used for all newborn babies at risk, as well as pre-term and term infants. It uses the manoeuvres of the NBAS in a graded sequence of increasingly vigorous stimuli from the environment, which can be interrupted as soon as they prove stressful for the baby. The assessment identifies:

- tasks handled with ease by the infant in the maintenance of well regulated and balanced functioning of all subsystems;
- tasks that are stressful and trespass the balance of the subsystems, but which can be handled with environmental support;
- tasks that are inappropriate for the infant at this stage.

Table 4.2   Withdrawal and approach behaviours.

Withdrawal
- Changes in heart rate, respiration, blood pressure, blood oxygenation, skin and toe temperature differential, pallor, mottling, greyness, cyanosis, jerks, startles, finger splay, toe splay, limb extension.
- Unco-ordinated movement, over-extension, hyper-hypotonus.
- Unco-ordinated sleep/wake cycle, persistent REM sleep, persistent irritability.
- Lack of eye contact, 'floating' eyes, facial expression of panic.
- Over-reaction to handling, no effort at self-consolation, no effort to regain comfortable position.

Approach
- Stable vital signs, synchronising skin and toe temperature, even colour, smooth movement, relaxed hands, willingness to grip finger.
- Relaxed position, good muscle tone.
- Maintenance of periods of deep sleep, periods of attentiveness (quiet/alert state).
- Direct gaze, alert look, turning of head or eyes to face or voice.
- Ability to return to sleep state on disturbance, sucking, rooting, hand-to-mouth movement, adapts body to positional change.

(Adapted from Als *et al.*, 1982.)

Assessment of Newborn Subsystem Development (ANSD)

The preterm infant will not be ready for social interaction until he has autonomic, motor and state control. To help him achieve this, the APIB and the model of synactive development have been summarised in a plan that demonstrates how the hospital environment may be adapted to fit the abilities of the individual infant (Sparshott, 1995b). By observing behaviour and adjusting environmental stimulation to obtain an optimal

Table 4.3 Assessment of Newborn Subsystem Development. Ability of the newborn infant to adapt to the hospital environment and adaptation of the hospital environment to the abilities of the newborn infant

Subsystems of functioning	Problem	Signs of instability	Possible interventions	Stability
Autonomic and physiological system Heart rate, respiration, blood pressure, temperature Colour Involuntary movement Digestive system	Immaturity or illness Pain Inappropriate environment Premature introduction to feeding	Changes in heart rate, respiration, blood pressure Skin and toe temperature differential Pallor, mottling, greyness, cyanosis Jerks, startles, finger splaying, limb extension Hiccoughs, spits, vomits, yawning, straining (as for bowel movement)	Treatment of illness Pain relief (analgesia or consolation) Comforting by 'containment' Gentle introduction of feeding Maintenance of safe environment	Stable vital signs Temperature synchronicity Even, pink colour Smooth movement Finger grip. or relaxed hands Tube feeds tolerated well Good sucking reflex Co-ordinated sucking
Motor system Posture Co-ordinated movement Muscle tone	Immaturity or illness Unsupported position Immobility Splinting	Over-extension, 'frog' position Unco-ordinated movement of limbs Range finding Hypertonus or hypotonus	Care of skin Support of limbs, maintenance of flexion, position changes, provision of barriers Padding and position of splint Stroking/massage	Flexed position Relaxed posture Good muscle tone 'Preening' or relaxing on stroking/massage
State system Sleeping and waking states (states of consciousness) – deep sleep, light sleep, drowsy, alert and awake, fussy crying, crying	Immaturity or illness Disturbance by: light, noise, repeated procedures, over-handling, different caregivers	Unco-ordinated sleep/wake cycle Persistent REM sleep Lack of deep sleep Persistent irritability	Provision of day/night cycle Protection from light and noise Respect of deep sleep state Regular periods of rest Grouping care Stimulation when ready Individualised care	Regular sleep/wake cycle Maintenance of periods of deep sleep Regular periods of attentiveness (quiet/alert state)

Table 4.3 Continued

Subsystems of functioning	Problem	Signs of instability	Possible interventions	Stability
Attentional/interactive system Reactions to face, voice and touch Reactions to taste and smell Response to animate and inanimate stimuli Response to immediate environment	Immaturity or illness Over-handling Lack of stimulation Separation from parents Lack of understanding by caregivers of behavioural cues	Lack of eye contact, floating eyes Only fleeting response to voice or touch Inability to maintain alert state Facial expression of panic Lack of 'cuddliness'	Stimulation by: eye-to-eye contact, talking or singing, calling to attention when in alert state Provision of cassettes/books Stimulation of senses (taste and smell) Parental presence	Periods of fixed attention Direct gaze, alert look Turning of head to face and voice Animated facial expression Bright expression, attempt at 'social smiling' Adapts body to caregiver
Self-regulatory system State control Self-quieting Avoidance behaviours Regulation manoeuvres	Immaturity or illness Over-handling Lack of understanding by caregivers of behavioural cues	Over-reaction to handling Inability to return to sleep state when awakened No effort at self-consolation No effort to regain comfortable position	Encouragement of self-regulation e.g. non-nutrative sucking, hand-to-mouth manoeuvre Respect of avoidance behaviour Stroking/massage	Ability to return to sleep state on disturbance Sucking, rooting, hand-to-mouth movement Adapts body to change of position

(From Sparshott, 1995b.)

Table 4.4   Chart for the Assessment of Newborn Subsystem Development.

Signs of instability	Signs of stability
(1) Autonomic system	**(1) Autonomic system**
Physiological signs	*Physiological signs*
Heart rate ☐☐ Respiration ☐☐	Heart rate regular ☐ Respiration regular ☐
Blood pressure ☐☐	Blood pressure regular ☐
Skin and toe temperature differential >1° ☐	Skin and toe temperature differential < 1° ☐
Colour	*Colour*
Pale ☐ Grey ☐ Mottled ☐	Smooth, even, normal colour ☐
Cyanosed ☐	
Involuntary movements	*Involuntary movements*
Jerks ☐ Startles ☐	Smooth ☐ Hand relaxed ☐
Finger splay ☐ Limb extension ☐	Finger grip ☐
Digestive system	*Digestive system*
Hiccoughs ☐ Spits ☐ Vomits ☐	Tube feeds tolerated ☐ Suck reflex ☐
Yawning ☐ Straining ☐	Co-ordinated sucking ☐
(2) Motor system	**(2) Motor system**
Frog position ☐	Flexed position ☐ Relaxed posture ☐
Unco-ordinated movement ☐	Good muscle tone ☐
Range finding ☐ Hypertonus ☐	'Preening' or relaxing on stroking/massage ☐
Hypotonus ☐	
(3) State system	**(3) State system**
Deep sleep ☐ REM sleep ☐	Regular sleep/wake cycle ☐
Awake/alert ☐ Fussy ☐	Sustained periods of deep sleep ☐
Crying ☐	Sustained periods of alertness ☐
	Smooth progression of states ☐
(4) Attentional/interactive system	**(4) Attentional/interactive system**
Avoidance of eye contact ☐	Sustained eye contact ☐
Only fleeting response to caregiver ☐	Animated facial expression ☐
Expression of panic ☐	Turning head to sound ☐
Floating eyes ☐	Turning head to object/face ☐
Lethargy/inattention ☐	Concentration on object/face ☐
	Attentional smiling ☐
(5) Self-regulatory system	**(5) Self-regulatory system**
Over-reaction to stimuli ☐	Ability to return to sleep state ☐
Lack of state control ☐	Hand-to-mouth movement ☐
No effort at self-consolation ☐	Adaption of body to position change ☐
No control of position ☐	Sucking/rooting ☐

(From Sparshott, 1995 b.)

response, caregivers are providing not only for the physical but also for the emotional and cognitive needs of the fragile baby.

The plan shows problems specific to each subsystem, and the signs of instability these are likely to provoke. Possible interventions are then followed by signs of stability so that caregivers may understand, by observing the infant's response, what consoling action is likely to be most effective (Table 4.3). The plan can be used in conjunction with a chart which should be completed at the end of each shift, showing how successful the caregiver has been in maintaining the baby in a state of stability (Table 4.4). Of course, failure may not be due to any fault on the part of the caregiver; it will also depend on the illness and fragility of the baby. Too many signs of instability can indicate, however, that further investigation is needed to find the cause of stress.

This plan, based on the APIB, is designed for practical use in a clinical setting. A detailed programme for the adjustment of the NICU environment to the individual infant is offered in the training programme of NIDCAP.

The Neonatal Individualized Developmental Care and Assessment Program (NIDCAP)

Disorganised behaviour of infants with bronchopulmonary dysplasia (BPD) may be modified by observation of behaviour and the use of strategies designed to comfort and console (Als *et al*, 1986). These strategies and the observation of behaviour from which they spring are the subject of a training programme for health care professionals offered at the Children's Hospital, Boston, and at other centres in the United States (Appendix 4). NIDCAP, which incorporates the APIB, is a formal education and training certification programme for health care professionals. Briefly, it is designed to provide a developmental approach to care so that caregivers can, through observation of infant behaviour and adjustment of working practices, provide a more supportive environment for the sick or preterm infant than purely technical skills can supply. In NICUs, 'infants are often receiving many varied levels of stimuli at once, which can be confusing and which cannot be integrated into meaningful learning experiences (VandenBerg, 1996). Studies into the beneficial effects of the NIDCAP have demonstrated not only improvement in developmental outcome as shown by significantly improved APIB scores, but also impressive cost savings.

The basic training programme takes place at two levels: Level I: Observational Training in Order to Improve Caregiving; and Level II: Formal Behavioral Assessment Training – APIB. Two more levels of training are necessary before trainees can themselves instruct others,

Table 4.5 Care plan for an infant of 28 to 32 weeks' g.a. in an incubator.

Date	Identified problem	Short-term goals	Nursing intervention
7/2	Alteration in state control due to prematurity and inappropriate environment	Nicole will have smooth transitions between states as evidenced by: (1) Heart rate and respiratory rate that remain within 10% of baseline during state transitions (2) Colour that remains pink during state transitions (3) Comes to drowsy then awake state rather than from sleep to agitation (4) Returns to sleep smoothly without autonomic instability or cycles of intense motor activity (5) Sleeps between caregiving sessions (6) Uses self-comforting behaviours such as: hand to mouth, foot bracing, or new strategies to self-regulate	Heavy cover over incubator to buffer light and sound stimuli Use of tape of parents' voices 10 minutes before hands-on caregiving to facilitate wake-up Provide hands-on head and lower extremities containment in silence for 15 seconds before interventions Assist infant to put her hands near her mouth and allow her to grasp caretaker's finger during caregiving Following caregiving, provide blanket rolls and snug 'envelope' to support her motor system Use lullaby tape provided by parents to help with transition back to sleep
7/30			Use of incubator cover over half to decrease amount of light Continued use of parents' voice tapes (varied) as infant wakens Offer of verbal greeting before beginning caregiving Continued support of self-regulation strategies, including new enjoyment of pacifier Following caregiving, provision of blanket roll support (she no longer needs 'envelope') Use of lullaby tapes only when she is fussy

(From Tribotti & Stein, 1992.)

and before a training centre for NIDCAP can be established. It is hoped to establish NIDCAP training centres in the UK; but this is yet to take place.

Evaluation of an infant using the APIB and NIDCAP can prove valuable as a basis for the planning and implementation of care by:

- the structuring of an infant's appropriate physical environment in the NICU;
- the timing and organisation of medical and nursing interventions;
- enhancing the parents' understanding of their infant as an individual;
- supporting parents in their confidence in specifically aiding their infant's development when confronting CNS compromise or chronic illness; and
- the work of special service providers such as early intervention programmes, public health nurses, physical therapists, etc., as they provide support for infant development after discharge from the NICU.

Table 4.5 shows how the NIDCAP can be used to create an individualised care plan for an infant of 28 to 32 weeks' g.a. in an incubator (Tribotti & Stein, 1992). The NIDCAP is lengthy, complex and expensive, but Tribotti and colleagues believe that its value in the prevention of major and minor sequelae in premature infants may outweigh these issues.

To implement NIDCAP, we need to be provided with a favourable basic environment. The structure of many NUs needs to be reconsidered; cramming as many incubators and ventilators as can be fitted into a large workshop will render individualised care impossible. In such places, stimulation to one means stimulation to all. What is the use of attempting to supply fragile babies with benign experiences of sound, if this will only add to the general cacophony? It cannot be right if caregivers are forced to suppress the comforting sounds of gentle music and voices, because the babies are already overwhelmed by the industrial sounds of intensive care. Hospital managers and architects need to bear this in mind when planning new units; inadequate provision for the emotional needs of fragile babies is a false economy.

Understanding preterm infant behaviour is not only important in order to create the most appropriate environment, it is essential in the promotion of a good relationship between parent and child. If parents can perceive their infant's inability to respond to them as a symptom of illness or immaturity rather than lack of interest, they can be encouraged to observe patiently improvements taking place over a passage of time.

Chapter 5
Infant Response to Pain and Distress

Acute, extreme and long lasting pain

Studies designed to reflect differences in behavioural and physiological response to invasive and non-invasive procedures have underlined the individuality of babies in their reactions to different stimuli (Grunau *et al.*, 1990); the response each baby makes will also depend on his gestational age, his physical condition, and his state of consciousness at that time (Sparshott, 1989a; 1994). The ability of a baby to control his own cycle of the states of consciousness is considered to indicate individual capacity for self-organisation and ability to adapt to environmental pressures; his reactions to trauma will therefore be influenced to a certain degree by his ongoing state.

Controversy exists as to whether the clinical responses of a newborn baby to noxious stimuli are due to 'pain' as perceived by an adult, or are merely reflex responses. Nonetheless, certain responses have come to be associated typically with acute, extreme and long lasting pain:

- *Acute pain* is highly localised, sharp and transitory, and subsides as healing takes place. It is experienced by the infant during the performance of traumatic procedures, when handled post-operatively, or spontaneously, in conditions such as colic.
- *Extreme pain* may be experienced in the performance of profoundly invasive procedures, such as the insertion of chest drains; or in illness such as necrotising enterocolitis (NEC), meningitis and glaucoma.
- *Chronic or long lasting pain* is intractable and persists over a period of time. In the newborn infant it includes recurrent acute pain such as is experienced through constant repetition of traumatic procedures; or persistent pain, as in such illnesses as NEC and cancer (Sparshott, 1989a, 1994).

Response to acute pain

There are certain behavioural responses and physiological changes that are associated with pain from invasive procedures:

- **Behavioural signs:** shown in vocalisation, facial expression and body movements.
- **Physiological changes:** seen in changes in heart rate, blood pressure, blood oxygenation, core and peripheral temperature differential, emotional sweating, and hormonal and metabolic changes.

Vocalisation

Crying, like feeding and sleeping, is a cyclical behaviour which is under neurophysiological control, but is also shaped by the environment (Messer *et al.*, 1993). Babies cry because they want something either to happen or to stop happening. Their distress may be due to hunger, a wet nappy, weariness, boredom or pain, but the message is always the same: 'Pay attention! I need help'. The signal given demands a response; it is up to the caregiver to interpret the signal and offer the appropriate satisfaction.

Even as every individual has a unique finger print, so babies can be identified by their crying (Wolff, 1969). Caregivers who spend a long time with their charges can usually recognise a baby by his cry. Their identification of its intention, however, may be influenced by the context; for instance, it is easy to assume that a child late for a feed cries from hunger – if he has been subjected to the procedure of heel-prick, however, the cry is more likely to be due to that painful experience.

The most commonly heard cry of the newborn infant is rhythmical; it may start suddenly, due to an external disturbance such as a loud noise or bright light, or it may progress from whimpering to the full blown demand to be fed. The cry of the hungry, uncomfortable baby usually starts with fussiness, and then builds up slowly, ceasing only when his needs are satisfied. The rapidity with which a mother responds to her baby will depend on the rhythm and intensity of the crying. Hearing the fussy cry, the mother may delay attending to her baby in order to finish a cup of tea; but if she stops for a second cup, her baby could cry himself into a state of tantrum from which he will be extricated with difficulty. By then, he may be exhausting himself by demonstrating the loud braying cry of the angry baby (Wolff, 1969).

Bowlby described the pain cry as:

> 'A sudden long and strong initial cry ... followed by a long period of absolute silence, due to apnoea: ultimately this gives way, and short gasping inhalations alternate with expiratory coughs' (Bowlby, 1969)

Wolff's similar description characterises a high pitched cry followed by a relatively long period without breathing, then a period of dysphonia gradually returning to the basic rhythmical cry (Wolff, 1969). Using *sound spectography* (the measurement of cry characteristics),

Michelsson *et al.* (1983) also found that pain-induced cries have a higher pitch than the main fundamental frequency; the first response being high-pitched but usually of short duration, followed by more normal low-pitched phonation. It is interesting to compare these three descriptions – the terminology is different, but all report the loud strong initial cry, then a short period of apnoea, followed by weaker wailing.

The highpitched initial cry was taken by Michelsson *et al.* to indicate the capacity of the CNS for controlled response. Lester and Zeskind (1982) also believed that the ability to organise cry in early infancy reflects the organisation of the CNS, and their studies indicated that even prenatal risk factors could affect the cry in a way related to behavioural organisation. If pain cry characteristics do reflect CNS stress, this is useful in the observation of healthy term infants; the high-pitched, piercing cry usually associated with cerebral irritation might also be produced as a reaction to acute pain. Sound spectography has also shown that the cries of sick full term and preterm babies tend to be more high-pitched than the cries of normal term infants (Michelsson *et al.*, 1983).

The general consensus of opinion, however, seems to be that there is no great difference between cry reactions to anger, hunger or pain, whether this is assessed by sound spectography or the human ear. The main differences between pain cries and the other types of cry lie in the fact that they sound louder and last longer (Gauvain-Piquard, 1989a; Grunau *et al.*, 1990); they do not indicate the *degree* of pain felt by the infant. But it is interesting to note that the urgent and intense cry which has been associated with pain is likely to compel the caregiver to come running, and that the shrill cry of the sick or preterm infant, impossible to ignore, will have the same effect; the so-called *pain cry* is an urgent demand which must be obeyed.

One more 'cry' remains to be described – this is the *silent cry* of the ventilated baby who can make no sound, but is seen to gape around the endotracheal tube (Wolke, 1987; Sparshott, 1989a) (Fig. 5.1).

Facial expression

Research undertaken by Grunau and Craig (1987) examined facial expression and cry in response to discomfort (heel-rub) and pain (heel-lance) as a function of four states of consciousness; the suggestion was that all responses to noxious stimuli would be moderated by the infant's ongoing state. The response to heel-rub was found to be substantially different from the constellation of changes observed following heel-lance, which were those demonstrated in the Neonatal Facial Coding System (NFCS) (Appendix 1): 'This reaction pattern may be described *operationally* as "pain" expression' (Grunau & Craig, 1987) (Fig. 5.2). The most marked differences were seen in oral responses; vertically

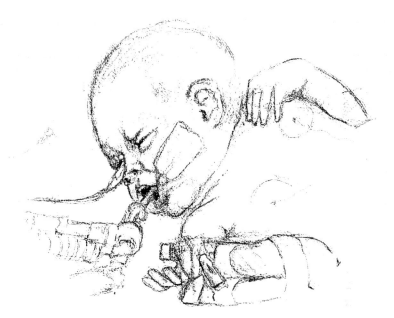

Fig. 5.1 The silent cry. (From Sparshott, 1994.)

stretched mouth and taut tongue: later, 'tongue protrusion' was added to the system, described as, 'Tongue visible between the lips extending beyond the mouth' (Craig & Grunau, 1993). Since it is of intrinsic importance to the survival of the newborn infant, oral function has always been taken to indicate the highest level of functional co-ordination.

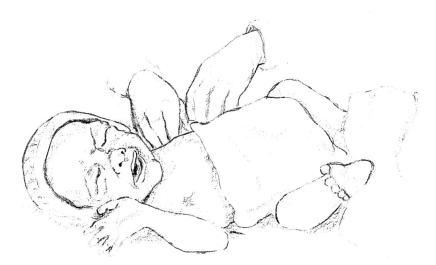

Fig. 5.2 Facial expression and body movement. (From Sparshott, 1994.)

Tissue damage was not the only factor determining the response of the newborn baby; pain expression was also found to be a function of ongoing behavioural state. The response of the babies disturbed during the 'quiet/awake' state differed from that of the babies in 'quiet' sleep (Fig. 5.3), supporting Brazelton's view that the baby is most receptive to environmental stimuli in the alert state. Differences in facial expression and cry across state seem to indicate the capacity of a healthy term baby to modify pain perception at an early age.

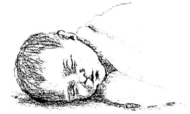

Quiet/sleep

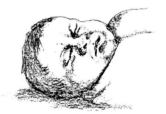

Heel-prick

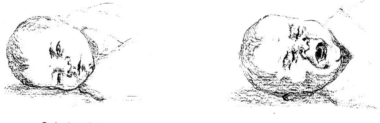

Quiet/awake   Heel-prick

Fig. 5.3   Facial behaviour in two babies. The upper row depicts an infant prior to heel-rub and the reaction to heel-lance during quiet/sleep. The bottom row depicts the reactions of a second infant during quiet/awake state. (From Sparshott, 1994, drawn from Grunau & Craig, 1987.)

Body movement

It is not as easy to read the motor signals of a baby as it is to understand crying or grimacing; movements frequently appear vague and undirected. However, a wide range of motor responses to traumatic stimuli have been identified, notably those described by McGraw (1941), Dale (1986) and Johnston and Strada (1986). Franck (1986) observed a two-component response of healthy term babies to heel-prick; immediate withdrawal of both limbs from the source of the injury, followed by crying. The crying was often accompanied by vigorous gross motor activity and grimacing, and movement of all extremities (Fig. 5.2); this two-part response seemed to support the contention that the infant experiences first and second pain as does an adult (Wachter-Shikora, 1981). In other words, the healthy term infant is capable of immediate motor response to painful stimuli (flight) followed by an emotional reaction (fright or fight).

Franck also noticed that the infants in her study seemed to respond less vigorously if they needed to be pricked a second time, and she suggests that squeezing the foot during the procedure may reduce, or at any rate change, the pain sensation, much as mechanical vibration, acupuncture and electric current may increase the pain threshold of adults by producing a counter irritant. In many cases, however, the more the foot is squeezed in order to obtain blood, the more violent the reaction is likely to be. Infants show great individuality in response to repeated heel-prick. Some will react with increased vigour each time, sometimes even crying and struggling as soon as the heel is touched, showing the function of short-term memory. Others who show a decreasing response may be becoming habituated to the sensation, and see no point in bestirring themselves.

Some babies show considerable co-ordination in response, such as 'side-swiping' at the site of injury with the other limb, or 'guarding' the source of pain with a cupped hand. But the very preterm infant, whose response to stimulus may be more vigorous than a term baby, is more likely to react with movements that are unco-ordinated, wild and diffuse. The great variety of motor responses to traumatic stimuli identified by researchers has been grouped by Craig *et al.* (1993) in the Infant Body Coding System (IBCS) (Appendix 1b).

Physiological changes

The physiological component of pain in infants can be observed in alterations in:

- heart rate
- blood pressure
- blood oxygenation
- central and peripheral temperature differential
- emotional sweating
- hormonal and metabolic changes.

Heart rate

Heart rate response to stimulus can be bi-directional; research has shown an increase in heart rate as a response to stress or fear, and a decrease as a response to mild visual and auditory stimulation (Owens, 1984). One would imagine from this that soothing voices and sweet music would cause the heart to slow down, and panic and pain would set it beating wildly, but with babies this does not always seem to be the case. Dale (1986) found that although the majority of infants in her study of body movement responded to pain with increased heart rate, two responded with deceleration. Williamson and Williamson (1983) found that during the cutting and clamping procedures of circumcision, some babies who had received local anaesthetic responded with such a deceleration of heart rate that it could be classed as bradycardia, whereas those who had not been anaesthetised showed an increase. Response to pain can therefore be seen in both increase and decrease in heart rate.

The reason for the slowing of the heart rate which sometimes seems to follow noxious stimulation may be due to the *valsalva* manoeuvre; when a baby cries, the increase in intrathoracic pressure causes a decrease in blood flow to the heart, leading to bradycardia (Brown, 1987). On the other hand, bradycardia is the most likely response of the fragile infant to stress. When considering responses to pain, then, alteration in heart rate can only be taken into consideration with other variables.

Blood pressure

Increase in blood pressure has been observed following heel-prick, during circumcision and during endotracheal suctioning, indicating an increase in cerebral blood flow and intracranial pressure (Perlman & Volpe, 1983; Williamson & Williamson, 1983; Brown, 1987).

Oxygenation

Decrease in $TcPO_2$ has been recorded during circumcision, tracheal intubation, suctioning, and following excessive handling in preterm infants (Long *et al.*, 1980; Williamson & Williamson, 1983); but increase is frequently seen in well term infants, particularly when crying (Wolke, 1987).

Temperature differential

Increase in central and peripheral temperature differential is taken to indicate a stress response in the sick or preterm infant, although this stress may be due to other causes than pain, notably infection, peripheral vasoconstriction due to hypovolaemia, the use of catecholamine infusions and drugs such as Dopamine, or even a wet nappy (Mitchell, 1996). Failure to maintain a normal central or core temperature due to cold stress will also, of course, result in a drop of peripheral temperature as the infant attempts to compensate. Temperature differential is significant, however, in a context where pain or distress are suspected, such as pain during venepuncture, or distress following overhandling by the caregiver (Mok *et al.*, 1991).

Emotional sweating

In contrast to the sweating that is due to a warm or humid environment and which is essential as a defence against overheating, emotional sweating from the palm of the hand and the sole of the foot is determined by emotional factors. Thermal sweating is controlled by the hypothalamus, while emotional sweating involves the higher centres in the cerebral cortex. It is increased by fear, anxiety and concentration, and decreased by contentment, relaxation and sleep. It has consequently been widely used in the study of stress responses; the lie detector is a well known example.

Emotional sweating from the palm of the hand occurs in newborn babies, sometimes as early as 36 weeks' g.a., regardless of gestation at birth, so that its development is largely unaffected by postnatal existence. In term babies it occurs on crying from the day of birth, and by the equivalent of 43 weeks' g.a. reaches levels comparable with those found in anxious adults (Harpin & Rutter, 1982).

Hormonal and metabolic changes

Studies in the hormonal activity in preterm and term babies undergoing surgery with minimal anaesthesia, as was at one time the practice, show that the subsequent release of corticosteroids and the suppression of insulin secretion lead to an increased metabolism of fat stores and carbohydrates, and prolonged periods of hyperglycaemia. These stress reactions are likely to last longer in preterm than in term infants, and are greater in magnitude than those of adult patients. Metabolic stress reaction is something the infant, with his limited stores of fat, protein and carbohydrate which he needs for growth, cognitive development and the assimilation of environmental stimuli, is ill-equipped to meet (Anand & Hickey, 1987).

Response to extreme pain

The extremity of pain felt is difficult to detect in the non-verbal infant, since neither study of facial expression nor spectographic analysis of crying can indicate the *intensity* of pain felt (Gauvain-Piquard, 1987). There are, however, certain abnormal positions of the limbs, and axial stiffness with the head thrown back, or the antalgic position of the body at rest, which may be indicative of intense suffering (the antalgic position is an unrelaxed, unnatural position adopted by the body as a defense against pain) (Fig. 5.4; Appendix 1c). The child with abdominal distention or meningitis who is in extreme pain will not be as easy to soothe as the infant who cries following heel-prick; he may calm himself for a moment when he is picked up and held, but as soon as he is replaced in his cot he will start to cry again – the pain continues, and will not have been magicked away.

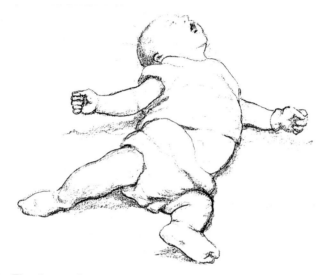

Fig. 5.4   The abnormal position of an infant in extreme pain. (From Sparshott, 1994, drawn from Gauvain-Piquard, 1987.)

When extreme pain is experienced the level of consciousness may diminish; this has been described as a 'sleeping fit' or 'coma vigil' (Burton & Derbyshire, 1958; Gauvain-Piquard, 1989a). Amongst other causes, severe pain should also be suspected in the infant who suddenly appears shocked, with grey pallor, lying limp and awake.

Response to long lasting pain

The baby in long lasting pain does not cry; it is impossible to cry for a long period of time without becoming exhausted, especially if the appeal meets with no response. He moves as little as possible in an attempt to economise energy and avoid further suffering; this immobility is said to resemble that of an animal faced with pain or danger. There is a failure to engage in communication with parents or caregivers; a reduction in alertness (the baby appears listless); and an expression of maturity, even hostility (Gauvain-Piquard, 1987). This is described as a mental and physical 'lack of tone', and because of its negativity, such a response is not easy to recognise:

> 'It is the picture of a child who appears sad, and who seems to have given up the fight ... movements of the limbs are slow and reluctant ... there is an appearance of dull hostility. These children turn their eyes away when approached, and take no initiative in a relationship.... A feeling of isolation and depression cannot be excluded.' (Gauvain-Piquard *et al.*, 1988)

Gauvain-Piquard is describing the non-verbal child, but experienced neonatal nurses will recognise the baby who, after weeks or months of illness and a constant bombardment of traumatic procedures, presents this picture of inertia, diminished alertness, withdrawal and hostility – very disconcerting to see in a baby (Appendix 1d). From the beginning, these infants have experienced a world where to be in pain is normal, and they have given up trying to defend themselves against it. Their resignation is such that caregivers frequently do not recognise the extent of their suffering. Attempts by a mother to elicit a response from a baby in chronic pain will be met with indifference; he may look away, apparently cold to her advances (Fig. 5.5). I have described such a baby in the introduction to this book; fortunately such infants are few, but they cannot be forgotten. There is a maturity, a look of mistrust, very like

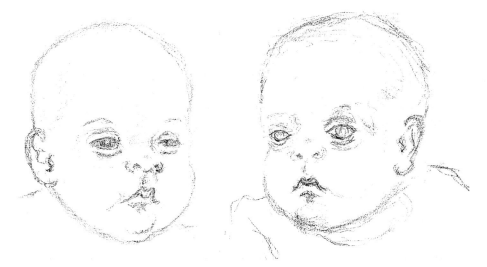

Fig. 5.5 Aaron – a very sick baby with BPD following prolonged ventilation and CPAP, showing eye avoidance and long lasting pain.

the expression of 'frozen watchfulness' described in the abused child, which is totally inappropriate in a newborn baby.

Pain scoring systems

The attempt to establish a scale to assess pain in the newborn is no new development. McGraw described neuromuscular responses of the newborn to noxious stimuli in 1941; in 1956 Graham *et al.* published a monograph describing behavioural differences between normal and traumatised newborn infants, using maturation, vision, irritability and tension. In 1986 Johnston and Strada offered a multidimensional description of acute pain response in infants. Gauvain-Piquard described reactions of the non-verbal child to extreme and long-lasting pain in 1987; this was adapted for use with the newborn by Sparshott in 1989 (Sparshott, 1989a; 1994).

More recently, Debillon incorporated the symptomatology of the newborn infant in pain into a score: this included facial expression; body movement; state of consciousness; method of communication (smile, cry, screaming); heart rate; oxygen saturation; and respiration (Debillon, 1992). In 1994, Bell demonstrated the use by neonatal nurses of a Postoperative Pain Score first developed by Attia *et al.* in 1987. This tool measures postoperative pain using degrees of behavioural response in: sleep; facial expression; spontaneous motor activity; response to ambient stimulation; flexion of fingers and toes; sucking; global evaluation of tone; consolability; and sociability.

Neonatal infant pain score (NIPS)

NIPS was a tool devised by Lawrence *et al.* (1993) to assess the behavioural reactions of preterm and full term babies to the painful stimulus of needle puncture. Operational definitions describe changes in facial expression, cry, breathing patterns, the movement of arms and legs, and state of arousal (Table 5.1). This is a validated scale, which the researchers suggest could be used in clinical trials and by experienced neonatal staff on the NICU, but they say: '... it cannot be used in isolation; the overall status of the infant and the infant's environment must be taken into account' (Lawrence *et al.*, 1993).

Distress Scale for Ventilated Newborn Infants (DSVNI)
(Appendix 2)

The DSVNI was devised to assess the physiological and behavioural responses of the ventilated newborn infant to any invasive procedure.

Table 5.1 NIPS operational definitions.

Facial expression
0 – Relaxed muscles	Restful face, neutral expression
1 – Grimace	Tight facial muscles, furrowed brow, chin, jaw (negative facial expression – nose, mouth and brow)

Cry
0 – No cry	Quiet, not crying
1 – Whimper	Mild moaning, intermittent
2 – Vigorous cry	Loud scream, rising, shrill, continuous. (*Note:* silent cry may be scored if baby is intubated, as evidenced by obvious mouth, facial movement)

Breathing patterns
0 – Relaxed	Usual pattern for this baby
1 – Change in breathing	Indrawing, irregular, faster than usual, gagging, breath holding

Arms
0 – Relaxed/restrained	No muscular rigidity, occasional random arm movement
1 – Flexed/extended	Tense, straight arms, rigid and/or rapid extension, flexion

Legs
0 – Relaxed/restrained	No muscular rigidity, occasional random leg movement
1 – Flexed/extended	Tense, straight legs, rigid and/or rapid extension, flexion

State of arousal
0 – Sleeping/awake	Quiet, peaceful, sleeping or alert and settled
1 – Fussy	Alert, restless and thrashing

ID #: _____ Procedure: _____

Name: _____ Date of procedure: _____

D.O.B.: _____ Procedure #: _____

Tape #: _____

	Before time		During time					After time		
	1	2	1	2	3	4	5	1	2	3
Facial expression 0 – Relaxed muscles 1 – Grimace										
Cry 0 – No cry 1 – Whimper 2 – Vigorous cry	1	2	1	2	3	4	5	1	2	3
Breathing patterns 0 – Relaxed 1 – Change in breathing	1	2	1	2	3	4	5	1	2	3
Arms 0 – Relaxed/restrained 1 – Flexed/extended	1	2	1	2	3	4	5	1	2	3
Legs 0 – Relaxed/restrained 1 – Flexed/extended	1	2	1	2	3	4	5	1	2	3
State of arousal 0 – Sleeping/awake 1 – Fussy	1	2	1	2	3	4	5	1	2	3
Total	1	2	1	2	3	4	5	1	2	3

(Time is measured in one (1) minute intervals)

(From Lawrence *et al.*, 1993.)

This scale includes the reactions of infants who have been subjected to repeated traumatic procedures, as well as immediate reactions to acute pain (Sparshott, 1996). Behavioural responses include degrees of facial expression, body movement and colour. Apart from the 'silent cry', differences in cry are not included in the scale as this response is not available to the ventilated baby. Examples of facial expression and body movement are accompanied by illustrations (Appendix 2, Table 3). The scale is based on the following scoring systems:

- The Neonatal Behavioral Assessment Scale (NBAS). (State of consciousness, colour.)
- The Assessment of Preterm Infant Behavior (APIB). (Facial expression, body movement, colour.)
- The Neonatal Facial Coding System (NFCS). (Facial expression: Appendix 1a.)
- The Infant Body Coding System (IBCS). (Body movement: Appendix 1b.)
- The Gustave-Roussy Child Pain Scale. (Extreme and long lasting pain: Appendix 1c and d.)

The DSVNI may be used for the assessment of babies of any gestational age, but it is not appropriate for infants demonstrating severe stress and 'shut down' through critical illness, or with neurological impairment, or who have been paralysed with pancuronium. Since perception as to what is painful differs from baby to baby, and the technical skill of caregivers is likely to vary, the type of traumatic procedure for which the score is used, and the number of attempts made, should be recorded (Appendix 2, Table 1). It would be impossible to describe and illustrate the multitude of expressions and movements available to each individual baby, but collective terminology (extension, flexion, etc.) can give an idea of the overall picture (Appendix 2, Table 2).

The scale for the assessment of facial expression and body movement is arranged for a score of 0–3, and 0–2 for colour; 0 normally, but not necessarily, being the baseline of the infant's state before being disturbed. Many ventilated infants may well be showing signs of distress before any procedure is performed; indeed, the cause of the distress may be the reason for the intervention. In this case, the baseline will of necessity be a higher score. Facial expression is classified as relaxed, anxious, anguished and inert. Body movements are classified as relaxed, restless, exaggerated and inert.

Physiological changes can be assessed from monitor readings of heart rate, blood pressure, oxygen saturation, and core and peripheral temperature differential; blood pressure can be omitted if a peripheral or umbilical line is not in place. Physiological signs should be read directly from the monitors (e.g. toe temperature: baseline: 36^2; during procedure:

35^8; after procedure: 35^2). Physiological changes are charted but not scored; their significance in relating to stress as distinct from illness will be in observed changes between baseline and post-trauma readings, and correlation between behavioural and physiological change. Colour changes are frequently more pronounced in the fragile, preterm infant who has no control over his central and autonomic nervous system. The infant who remains pale, mottled or grey throughout the procedure is likely to be demonstrating an autonomic system that is already stressed. It must be remembered that it may be difficult to assess skin changes in infants from races with deep pigmentation of the skin.

Four recordings are taken: one before, one during, and two following the procedure. The pre-procedure recording is taken as a baseline even if the infant already shows stress. The second reading is the immediate response of the baby to the trauma. The third recording should be made approximately three minutes after the procedure, or as soon as the caregiver has re-positioned the baby. If at this time the baby cannot be consoled, it should enable the caregiver to distinguish between the 'anguished' and 'exaggerated' responses of the infant immediately following an extremely painful procedure, and the same responses persisting in the infant who continues in extreme pain (i.e. following chest drain insertion). The fourth score should be recorded after one hour, which gives the caregiver time to comfort and console the baby, or administer analgesia if necessary. Study of all scores should show the caregiver not only to what degree the baby has been distressed, but also whether she has succeeded in returning the baby to a state of equilibrium. A guide to score assessment is shown in Appendix 2.

Scores may not necessarily indicate identical behaviour; for example, the term baby may respond to a sharp, acute pain with Score 2 'anguished' facial expression and Score 1 'restless' body movements, whereas the very preterm infant is more likely to respond to the same stimulus with Score 1 'anxious' and Score 2 'exaggerated'. It is expected that the infant suffering the effects of long lasting pain will show Score 3 'inert' response in both facial expression and body movement. The aim is to keep the intermediate scores low, and for the final score to be 0 ('relaxed'), or at least back to baseline. One more important item needs to be noted, and that is the time it takes for the baby to return to baseline; duration of response and recovery are indicative of the recuperative powers of the baby, and the successful consoling techniques of the caregiver.

The DSVNI is designed to assess the responses of ventilated babies, who of all infants in hospital are the most subjected to invasive procedures. The behavioural stress responses of ventilated babies are more likely to be pronounced owing to their fragility and/or prematurity; infants requiring intensive care are more likely to have monitoring systems in place, which renders physiological changes easier to record. There is no reason, however, why the behavioural score of the DSVNI cannot be used by caregivers for the assessment of any newborn infant subjected to a traumatic procedure, even if the absence of monitoring makes recording physiological changes impractical; most of the behavioural reactions, if not their significance, will already be recognisable by experienced neonatal nurses.

Changes in physiological signs, colour, and indeed many of the behavioural characteristics, can of course be brought about by many different sources of stress; however, these changes taken all together, and in situations where traumatic procedures are performed, are most likely to indicate distress due to pain.

Some differences in behaviour are subtle, and require experience and knowledge of the individual baby on the part of the caregiver. The random, unco-ordinated movements of the preterm infant who has not been assailed should not be confused with the thrashing and flailing of the infant reacting to venepuncture; splaying, or 'starring', of the fingers may be a simple stretching movement if it is not associated with other 'exaggerated' responses. On the other hand, 'exaggerated' responses might well be associated with the infant protesting against inappropriate ventilator settings, rather than an immediate response to acute pain. *Context* and *duration* are the important factors.

Note: it would be very dangerous to assume that inertia must be due to pain; such a response might be seen in extreme illness, brain damage, or in certain congenital disorders. Nor is it likely to be the reaction to pain of the ventilated preterm infant. The baby who presents this response (or lack of it) has usually been in intensive care a long time, such as the baby with chronic respiratory problems who cannot be weaned from the ventilator. It presents as an apparent indifference to trauma, and is characterised by a refusal to react during or after a traumatic procedure. It is the response of the baby who has learnt that responding does not matter – again, the *context* is important.

The DSVNI is research based and should be capable of demonstrating the severity of distress experienced by an individual baby during and following a traumatic procedure; it is quick to apply, and can be used in routine clinical practice.

Part II
The Invasive Environment

Chapter 6
Pain and Therapy

Categories of environmental disturbance

While the basic physiological necessities for living are catered for in the NICU by the life support systems, there are other fundamental needs that are not supplied by them. These emotional requirements are perhaps not essential for life (though this is debatable), but they are certainly necessary for development – a 'home' must be created for the baby within the hospital environment which will supplement emotional as well as physiological deprivation (Fig. 1 in the Introduction; Sparshott, 1990). Since the infant is not yet able to adjust to the environment, the caretaking environment must adjust to the infant's capacities, and give support.

The adverse experiences of the newborn baby in hospital can be divided into three categories: those caused by pain, discomfort and disturbance. Against these can be set the beneficial actions of treatment, consolation and cherishment (Table 6.1; Sparshott, 1991c; 1994). Many of these experiences are interchangeable, depending on the individual baby, his g.a., physical condition, and state of consciousness. What may be perceived by one baby as painful, as expressed by behaviour and physiological changes, may be merely uncomfortable for another, and actions taken to alleviate the distress will depend on the caregiver's perception of the baby's perceptions. The baby's response to the actions we take will show us whether we have judged rightly.

Much can be achieved if caregivers are sensitive to the effect the hospital environment may have on an individual baby, whether term or preterm. An intrusive environment can cause distress; in Part II of this book, we will discuss ways of adapting the environment to the needs of infant and caregiver.

Traumatic procedures: whether necessary and when

The more often traumatic procedures need to be repeated, the more the infant will be distressed, and the longer he will take to recover; expertise

Table 6.1   Categories of environmental disturbance and their treatment.

Pain	Discomfort	Disturbance
Intubation	Monitoring	Light
Chest drain insertion and removal	Physical examination	Noise
	Extubation	Cold
Venepuncture	Range finding, due to insecurity	Heat
Heel-prick		Nappy change
Suctioning	Chest physiotherapy	Position change
I.m. injection	Electrode removal	Nakedness
Wound cleansing	Rectal temperature	Weighing
CPAP	Passage of NG or OG-tube	Overhandling
Lumbar puncture	I.v. medication	Feeding by NG or OG tube
Arterial or suprapubic stab	Splinting	Bottle feeding when too weak
Surgery	Physical restraint	
Illness, e.g. meningitis, necrotizing enterocolitis	Phototherapy	Isolation
	Urine bag removal	Separation
	Adhesive tape removal	Lack of stimulation if well
	Hunger	Noxious taste/odour

Therapy	Consolation	Cherishment
Prevent pain by:	Music and sound	Day and night lighting
Technique	Provision of boundaries	Noise reduction
Preparation beforehand	Containment	Minimal handling or stimulation
Choice of equipment	Stroking and massage	
Abstention	Swaddling	Clothing and coverings
Grouping care	Rocking	Parental presence
Treat pain by:	Non-nutritive sucking	Soft toys
Analgesia	Breastfeeding	Musical toys and cassettes
Local anaesthetic	Encouragement of self-consolation (hand-to-mouth movement)	Pictures
Anaesthetic cream		Mirrors
Treat intractable pain by:		Mobiles
Relief of symptoms	Encasement	Baby carriers
Containment	Correct positioning	Baby chairs
Narcotic analgesia		Skin-to-skin contact
		Pleasant taste/odour

(From Sparshott, 1994.)

and a good technique are therefore essential. There should be no illusions; all traumatic procedures, no matter how perfectly done, are going to hurt the baby to some degree. There is no reason, however, why we should not try to limit the damage we do as much as we can.

Before considering ways of treating the pain and consoling the baby, neonatal staff should ask themselves certain questions:

(1)   Is the action really necessary?

For instance, lumbar puncture is usually included in routine screens for infection. Lumbar puncture is a valuable diagnostic tool, but it is also painful and potentially dangerous (McGrath & Unruh, 1987). It is difficult to perform and only too often skin perforation needs to be repeated when undertaken by an inexperienced practitioner; should it not, therefore, only be performed when absolutely necessary, and not at all if the information required can be gained by other means?

(2) The action is necessary – but must it be taken now?

Routine blood samples are generally taken by Senior House Officers (SHOs) in the course of daily duties, and they will therefore 'go round' the babies in order to complete their tasks methodically. The baby with sleeping problems may well be disturbed at the moment he most needs to be left to rest. In this case, would it not be better to allow the infant his much needed sleep than to satisfy the demands of the laboratory, or the conscience of the doctor about to finish the shift? If the demands of the baby were really placed first, the accomplishment of a routine task at a certain time might not be so vitally important.

(3) The action is necessary – but can it be combined with any other?

Collaboration between doctors and nurses is essential; they can combine blood sampling, so that the baby does not have to be hurt twice. Fragile babies will profit from 'grouping' care, when the performance of a painful procedure can be followed by basic care (such as a positional or nappy change) which will allow the nurse to comfort the baby, and which can be followed by a period of absolute calm. Here, as always, the reactions of the individual baby need to be taken into account. Routine nursing care should not take precedence over minimal handling if the baby shows signs of stress – he should be left, in a comfortably supported position, to recover.

Nursing care plans for pain management

Saving time (without sacrificing safety) is a priority for nurses who are caring for ill babies in the NICU. Detailed care plans for pain management and pain scores are useful as references or for teaching purposes, but in the clinical field they must be functional, or nurses will have neither the time nor the patience to use them. Nurses often feel that with too many charts to complete and reports to write they are kept from their primary objective, which is the care of the baby; but if no written record is made of the individual baby's reactions to pain, it will be only too easy to ignore them. The only way to demonstrate that a baby is suffering from the ill effects of trauma is to show it to be so; the nurse is then in a much better position to be the baby's advocate and intervene.

The *objectives* of a care plan are to individualise nursing care, help the nurse sort out priorities and develop a problem solving approach to patient care, and to aid in communication between all members of the health care team (McFarlane & Casteldine, 1982). The *value* of a care plan lies not in its complexity but in its simplicity, since a care plan should be designed for practical use.

Wolke (1987) suggests that three principles are involved in structuring an individualised care plan for a baby. These are:

(1) to observe the baby before, during and after a traumatic procedure, and to note his reactions to handling, sound and light;
(2) on the basis of these observations, to form a plan with the health team to minimise the effects of stress, and support development and the organisation of behaviour;
(3) to adapt this plan as the baby progresses.

Ideally, these principles could be adapted and combined by the NU staff in a shared responsibility with parents – nurses can draw up a plan recording emotional and physiological responses, and parents can suggest how best, in their experience, their baby may be kept in a state of well-being (see Chapter 9; Fig. 9.1). Parents are often quick to notice any changes in the behaviour of their child, for they are beside him every day, and their concern (and therefore their concentration) is great.

Several nursing care plans have been published which show behavioural responses and developmental interventions (Cole & Frappier, 1985; Lawhon, 1986; Franck, 1989). The 'Plan of care for pain management in the special care baby unit (SCBU)' (Table 6.2; Sparshott, 1989a; 1994) is specifically designed to record reactions to pain due to traumatic procedures, surgery and illness. It includes:

● observations of state of consciousness and physiological signs made before, during and after a traumatic procedure;
● the type of procedure and the length of time it takes to perform;
● what actions are taken to soothe the baby and whether analgesia is necessary; and
● how long it takes to restore the baby to a state of equilibrium.

To help achieve these goals, a chart may be kept to record observations which, once the coding system has been grasped, requires only 'ticks', and the recording of vital signs if monitoring systems are in place (Table 6.3).

Table 6.2 Plan of care for pain management in the SCBU.

Problem	Goal	Nursing intervention	Nursing Evaluation

Pain from: Traumatic procedures	Prevention of unnecessary suffering
	
	Maintenance of a safe environment
	
	Restoration to a state of equilibrium
		(1) Observe:
		  • state of consciousness
		  • physiological signs prior to procedure
		(2) Perform or assist with procedure:
		  • causing as little disturbance to baby as possible
		  • maintaining safe environment by keeping baby warm and in most comfortable position
		  • suggesting administration of local anaesthetic if appropriate
		(3) Note time taken over procedure
		(4) Note immediate behavioural and physiological response
		(5) Comfort and console baby until calm once procedure is completed
		(6) Suggest administration of analgesia if necessary
		(7) Observe state of baby and physiological changes
		(8) Note time taken and methods used to restore baby to a state of equilibrium
			Goal is achieved when baby is restored to state of equilibrium: the shorter the time, the greater the success of the nursing intervention

Post-surgery	As above	(1) Anticipate that pain will be experienced
		(2) Ensure that appropriate analgesia has been prescribed
		(3) Observe for signs of pain
		(4) Take appropriate action by:
		  • alleviating symptoms
		  • administration of analgesia
		(5) Observe state of baby and physiological changes
		(6) Note time taken and methods used to restore baby to a state of equilibrium
			As above

Illness Extreme and lasting pain	As above	As in post-surgery	As above

Note: observations of state, maintenance of safe environment and attempts to comfort and console should be made in all cases.
(From Sparshott, 1989a. Reproduced by kind permission of *Nursing Times* where first published 11 October 1989.)

Table 6.3 Chart for recordings before, during and after a traumatic procedure.

Date and time														
State before procedure Asleep														
Awake														
Crying														
Heart rate*														
Respiration														
Blood pressure*														
TcPO$_2$ (or O$_2$ sat.)*														
Procedure Time taken (minutes)														
Reaction														
Nursing action Voice														
Stroking														
Massage														
Cuddle														
Rocking														
Swaddle														
Non-nutritive sucking														
Breast/bottle feeding														
Containment														
Analgesia														
Other														
Result Asleep														
Awake														
Crying														
Heart rate*														
Respiration														
Blood pressure*														
TcPO$_2$ (or O$_2$ sat.)*														
Achieved 1 – 3 minutes														
3 – 5 minutes														
5 – 10 minutes														

Code

Invasive procedures		*Expected reactions*	
CD	Insertion of chest drain	C	Cry
LP	Lumbar puncture	FE	Facial expression (grimace)
INT	Intubation	BM	Body movement
ETS	Endotracheal suctioning	Nil	No response
VP	Venepuncture		
AS	Arterial stab		
HP	Heel-prick		
	(Other)		

*These observations need only be made if monitoring equipment is already in place; otherwise even more disturbance will be caused to the baby.

(From Sparshott, 1989a, reproduced by kind permission of *Nursing Times* where first published on 11 October 1989.)

Traumatic procedures: how?

It would take too long to discuss all the invasive procedures infants must undergo in the NU, especially as technology and (consequently) techniques are changing all the time; but examination of some of the most common and most traumatic procedures may help to give some idea of ways in which caregivers can minimise the distress they cause.

Ventilation

The endotracheal (ET) tube for mechanical ventilation, whether passed through the mouth or nostril, must be fixed so that it cannot be dislodged. Movement of the tube may not only be painful, it can also cause local trauma to the larynx, and a deterioration in condition due to stimulation of the vagus nerve. The tube must be the right size; too small a gauge may pass beyond the vocal cords and cause trauma to the larynx. Since too much movement can easily dislodge the tube, the baby's head must be supported in such a way as to give security, without restricting blood flow or causing constraint.

'Awake' intubation has been shown to produce higher intra-cranial pressure in babies who have not been sedated; anaesthetised intubation will reduce this risk and eliminate pain during the delicate procedure of passing the tube (Yaster, 1987). Of course this may not be possible if the intubation is performed as an emergency; speed and safety come first.

The selection of the most appropriate ventilator settings is important for the baby subjected to Continuous or Intermittent Mandatory Ventilation (CMV/IMV). Considerable distress can be experienced by an infant who tries to breathe against the ventilator. If adjusting the ventilator settings has no effect, 'fighting' the ventilator can be prevented by paralysing the baby with pancuronium given intravenously. The infant may use the 'exaggerated' motor responses of the DSVNI in his struggle with the ventilator (Appendix 2, Tables 2 and 3) – but once paralysed he has no way of demonstrating his discomfort. To prevent unnecessary suffering, therefore, it is preferable that an analgesic infusion should be given routinely with pancuronium. The introduction of patient triggered ventilation (PTV), which allows the baby to breathe at his own rate, has reduced the necessity for using paralysing drugs. PTV appears to be less stressful than conventional methods of ventilation for the preterm infant (Greenough & Greenall, 1988); this is currently the subject of a trial, the results of which are not yet known.

The magnitude of distress caused to the infant during extra-corporeal membrane oxygenation (ECMO), high frequency oscillation and other methods of ET ventilation is unclear; but sedation is usually considered during these procedures.

Continuous positive airways pressure (CPAP)

CPAP is usually administered by means of single or double nasal prongs or a tube passed through one nostril. As a transition from full ventilation to independence, its value is indubitable, but the system can cause problems.

The baby promoted to CPAP is usually no longer critically ill, and may well be irritable and restless. If the pressure is administered by nasal tube, he is likely to be uncomfortable and may attempt to dislodge it by shaking his head; the more he struggles to be rid of the tube, the more it will irritate, causing friction to sensitive mucosa. The baby may be difficult to feed because of air passing into the stomach, which will necessitate the passage of a naso-gastric tube through the other nostril to prevent gastric distention; if care is not taken, the nostrils can become so traumatised that stenosis of the nasal passages results. Moistening or lubricating the tube can be helpful, and some NUs use lignocaine gel to deaden sensation around the nostrils, but care must be taken not to block the tube. Lignocaine gel can only be used externally, so it does not relieve pain from trauma to nasal mucosa.

Nasal prongs used with a CPAP flow driver, if the right size are selected and if they fit snugly, appear to be less traumatic than the nasal tube. If the infant is very restless and distressed and fails to settle (and if he is sufficiently mature), a sedative such as chloral hydrate can be used to prevent him inflicting damage on himself. Chloral hydrate is useful for the short-term treatment of insomnia and restlessness, but it has no pain relieving properties. It can cause excitement and gastric irritation, so should only be given in conjunction with feeding. Prolonged use can also cause renal damage.

Suctioning

There are two methods of suctioning: deep and shallow. Deep suctioning can lead to perforation of segmental bronchi, pneumothorax and pneumomediastinum; it may, however, be necessary for the baby with copious secretions. Shallow suctioning is less traumatic but predisposes to tube blockage, resulting in emergency re-intubation. Frequent re-intubation, besides being painful, can lead to laryngeal damage varying from oedema and pseudo-membranes to tracheal and subglottal stenosis. For the baby with minimal secretions, however, shallow suctioning should be adequate to keep the airway clear (Kleiber, 1986).

Suctioning pressure should be between 50 and 100 cm/H_2O (or as little as is necessary to clear the airway) to prevent damage to the oropharyngeal mucosa. Catheters should not pass beyond the end of the ET tube, so the tube should be measured; if a tape showing the length of the tube is fastened to the top of the incubator, the nurse can measure the suction catheter against this and thus avoid going in too far. The end of the catheter should always be withdrawn 1–2 cm if it comes up against the mucosa. If secretions are dry and resistant, the catheter can be lubricated with distilled water or with lignocaine gel, but, again, care must be taken not to block the airway. 0.1–0.2 ml/kg of sterile sodium chloride 0.9% injected into the endotracheal tube or the nostril may help soften the secretions, but should only be instilled just before suction to enhance retrieval of the solution (Kleiber, 1986; Hodge, 1991; Young, 1995). Some researchers, however, believe that if the ventilation is adequately humidified, irrigation of the airway should not be necessary, and may in fact be detrimental (Shorten *et al.*, 1991; Hodge, 1991; Wilson *et al.*, 1992).

ET suctioning leads to hypoxia, a drop in heart rate, increased blood pressure and increased cerebral blood flow (Wolke, 1987); it causes a greater instance of drop in blood oxygenation than either changing the baby's position or heel-prick blood sampling. It has been shown that babies suffer less hypoxia when nurses modify their suctioning techniques by limiting the time of the procedure or allowing the baby to rest when stressed (Beaver, 1987). Suctioning should be performed as expeditiously as possible, therefore, and reduced to the minimum necessary for safety.

Chest drain insertion

The insertion of chest drains through the chest wall is usually performed as an emergency treatment for pneumothorax, which means that the medical team have to act quickly. Nonetheless, this is an extremely painful procedure, and the baby will be put at risk if analgesia or local anaesthetic has not been administered; a baby can collapse into a state of shock following such treatment. The administration of a bolus dose of morphine beforehand, and the preparation of the site by means of local anaesthetic, is indispensable if the baby is not to be subjected to extreme pain.

It must not be forgotten that, once in place, the chest drain remains in an open wound. The infant will be spared a continuation of the pain by the administration of an analgesic infusion, and by the correct fixing and support of the drain to prevent any dragging on the infant's chest wall. For the same reason, great care should be taken when the infant's position is changed; preferably two nurses should be present for greater control.

It should also be remembered that the removal of a chest drain is painful, and appropriate analgesia will be necessary before such a procedure.

Venepuncture/line placement

Venepuncture is a procedure the success of which depends on the skill of the caregiver. The preterm infant may require i.v. nutrition for a long period of time, and since immature veins are fragile and difficult to find, particularly if the infant is hypovolaemic, frequent resiting of cannulae may be necessary.

The most suitable superficial veins for i.v. infusion are in the antecubital fossa, the back of the hand, the top of the foot, the long saphenous at the ankle, and the scalp (Whitelaw & Valman, 1980; Roberton, 1986). A good light is essential to work in, and while the cannula is being inserted another person should hold and comfort the baby, or give him an opportunity for non-nutritive sucking.

Scalp veins, once the cannula is in place, are said to be painless; caregivers must invent a way to protect the area while allowing for observation and the passage of the i.v. line. This can be done by using a gallipot with one small section cut out for the passage of the line, and another to allow for observation of the site of the needle tip (Fig. 6.1); but the cut-out section must be trimmed to prevent pressure of sharp edges on the scalp. The area must be shaved first, which is distressing for parents, and they should be reassured that the hair will grow again. The forehead should be avoided, as extravasation of hypertonic fluids or calcium will leave scars (Whitelaw & Valman, 1980). If extravasation does occur, the immediate application of a small amount of Percutol locally will help prevent permanent scarring. Glyceryl trinitrate 2% ointment is used in this case to reduce inflammation and stimulate circulation; it has no analgesic properties.

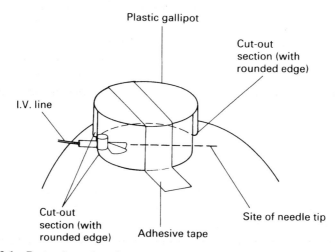

Fig. 6.1 Protection of scalp-vein site. (Adapted from Whitelaw & Valman, 1980.)

For the newborn baby who needs frequent blood sampling, umbilical arterial catheterisation can be used, which (as far as one knows) once established is not painful. When parenteral nutrition needs to be given over a long period of time, the insertion of a central line may avoid the constant resiting of peripheral lines; this needs skill to install and a high degree of supervision and hygiene to manage safely. Parenteral nutrition and antibiotics can be administered by a peripheral line, while at the same time an arterial line, using a solution of heparinised saline, can be used to obtain blood samples; this will obviate the need for repeated heel-pricks.

The insertion of an i.v. cannula requires skill and a good technique (Whitelaw & Valman, 1980); SHOs and neonatal nurses must acquire this through practice. The caregiver installing the cannula must remember that, quite apart from increasing the infant's distress, repeated failure to find a vein leads to spoiling veins for others. The nurse, as the baby's advocate, should make sure that after a third failed attempt, or even before if the infant shows signs of extreme distress, more expert help is sought; and in the case of the critically ill baby whose stability is already compromised, expert help should be sought straight away.

Subcutaneous local anaesthetic can be used to prevent pain during venepuncture, but since this is also administered with a needle its value is debatable. Anaesthetic creams are administered topically to produce anaesthesia of the skin, and are non-traumatic; Emla cream (lignocaine base 25 mg and prilocaine base 25 mg) has been used successfully to reduce pain from such procedures as heel-prick and venous cannulation (Maunuksela & Korpela, 1986; Fitzgerald *et al.*, 1989; Abajian & Sethna, 1993). The disadvantages are: it needs to be applied *at least* one hour before the performance of a traumatic procedure; it can only be used in very small quantities so the exact site of application must be known; and the effect of absorption through infant skin is uncertain.

In order to avoid the trauma of i.m. administration of antibiotics, an indwelling cannula is usually left in situ and kept patent by regular flushes of sodium chloride 0.9%. Since babies receiving antibiotics in this manner are usually active and vigorous, the cannula must be well secured.

Heel-prick

Heel-prick for the collection of blood is routinely performed on babies on post-natal and children's wards as well as the NU, so all midwives and nurses are likely to become familiar with the technique.

To avoid tissue atrophy, the formation of painful cysts, and osteomyelitis of the *os calcis*, heel-pricks should be performed on the plantar surface of the heel, beyond the lateral and medial limits of the *calcaneus*

(Roberton, 1986). From these small areas of the heels blood samples can be taken for tests which require only small volumes of blood. The method used is to prick the baby's heel using a small lancet and to squeeze gently until a drop of blood is formed (Fig. 6.2). Warming the heel beforehand will help promote blood flow in infants who do not bleed easily, and rubbing a little lanolin on the site will help in the formation of a drop of blood. Over-enthusiastic squeezing of the heel not only causes pain but also damages tissue.

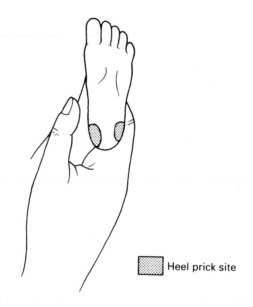

Heel prick site

Fig. 6.2 Heel-prick blood sampling. (Adapted from Whitelaw & Valman, 1980.)

The automated incision device (a number of models are now available) is a mechanical device specially designed for capillary blood sampling. It consists of a stylet held in a spring-loaded cartridge which is placed against the skin of the heel. When released by the cartridge, the stylet pierces the skin to a depth of 2.4 mm and is immediately withdrawn. This device is seen to be a safer method of obtaining blood samples than the lancet, which, since it is impossible to control, might give an incision depth varying from 1.4 mm to 3.0 mm, thereby increasing the risk of heel damage (Harpin & Rutter, 1983; McGrath & Unruh, 1987; Blain-Lewis, 1992).

Understanding the infant's state of consciousness can be useful. It is sometimes possible to take a heel-prick blood sample from a well term baby during a period of deep sleep and provoke very little response; if the baby's position is not disturbed, and if the heel-prick is done quickly, lightly and once only, the baby may hardly stir, and will immediately settle into sleep again (Fig. 5.3) (Grunau & Craig, 1987; Sparshott, 1989a; 1994). This is less likely to occur if the procedure has to be repeated, or if the pain is intensified by squeezing the heel; nor will it be possible in the case of the fragile or preterm infant, who cannot co-ordinate states. Obviously, it would not be good practice to risk interrupting the deep sleep of the baby who already has sleeping problems.

Lumbar puncture

Lumbar puncture is often included in routine infection screens, but it is both painful and uncomfortable and, unless it is unsafe to do so, should be avoided (McGrath & Unruh, 1987). As in venepuncture, the success of the procedure depends on a good technique, and in the case of failure should not be repeated more than twice; attempts should be discontinued if the baby shows signs of distress.

To obtain entry into the spinal cord, the infant must be grasped and held in a bow position, head to knees; too tight a grasp and too extreme a curve may block the airway, and the baby will resist, making the procedure more difficult. The baby should be moved into position slowly and gently, the hold should be firm but not tight, and the caregiver should talk soothingly to the baby while the procedure is performed. Sometimes a soft rolled towel or blanket tucked against the abdomen for the baby to curl round will help him feel less insecure. Since the baby is exposed, he will need to be protected from the cold by adjusting the incubator or room temperature beforehand, and by keeping his body covered as much as possible without impeding the procedure. He should not be left, after the procedure, until he has been settled comfortably once more.

Local anaesthetic can be administered before lumbar puncture, but this involves the use of yet another needle. Emla cream is sometimes used, at the discretion of the doctor, to provide topical anaesthesia of the skin.

Treatment of extreme and long lasting pain

The relief offered to the infant in *extreme pain* will depend partly on the cause of the pain. Diagnosis must be followed by appropriate action; for instance, relief of abdominal distention for the infant with necrotising enterocolitis, protection from sound and light in meningitis, soothing local applications and dressings in the treatment of burns. These actions will not be sufficient by themselves, and should always be supported by analgesia.

Parents find it hard to watch their baby reacting with violence to suffering. Their instinct is to hug him, rock him and caress him. The infant in extreme pain may calm for the moment in the arms of his parents, but this will not last long; stimulation at the moment of a paroxysm of pain may even increase the sensation, and the infant may present, besides an unnatural position (see Appendices 1c and 2, Tables 2 and 3), all the signs of stress due to intense internal or external stimuli. Consolation techniques are not likely to help the baby in extreme pain; he needs to be moved as little as possible, lying with limbs supported in his preferred position. However, in the case of an infant who can bear to be touched, it might be possible to offer some consolation by means of containment or encasement (Als, 1986; Sparshott, 1994).

Containment may be considered a method of consolation which is suitable for the fragile infant who reacts unfavourably to stroking, since it involves physical contact but is essentially passive. The infant is 'encased' in the incubator by the provision of steady boundaries in the form of rolled blankets against his sides and the soles of his feet; one hand of the caregiver is placed over the crown of his head, the other over his trunk. He is then 'contained' by the hands and gently and lightly held, without stroking, a manoeuvre which demands no response (Fig. 6.3). When the baby is in a sufficiently alert state for the caregiver to initiate social contact, this must be begun slowly, with the caregiver holding him, looking at him and slightly smiling, but still without trying to catch

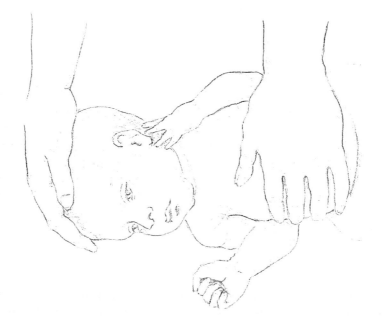

Fig. 6.3 'Containment'.

his attention (Als, 1986). Als suggests that stimulation can be added starting with eye contact alone, without talking. It must be remembered, however, that the NICU is never silent; stimulation from extraneous mechanical sounds cannot be avoided. To counteract this, in my experience, even very fragile infants will be comforted by and respond to the soft tones of a human voice. As with all procedures, the success of these manoeuvres can be judged by the physiological and emotional response of the baby.

The baby in *chronic pain* needs minimal handling, protection from light and noise, and the support of analgesia. If tactile consolation is attempted, containment is an action that parents can take, and may help them to feel less frustrated by their inability to help protect their baby from pain; they too can learn whether they have been successful by watching the responses of the baby. But even containment may be too much for the baby at first. The time for love and cherishing will come when analgesia begins to take effect and the pain abates – undemanding love is needed for babies in chronic pain.

Obviously, all unresponsive, inert babies will not necessarily be suffering from pain – it would be dangerous to assume so; other physiological or congenital conditions will need to be investigated. If the caregiver suspects, however, from knowledge of the baby and his history, or from observation of his behaviour, that in the context pain could be the cause of his comportment, she should take steps to see that appropriate analgesia is prescribed.

Use of analgesia

Opinions differ on which narcotic and analgesic drugs are most suitable for treatment of the newborn. While underlining the importance of providing adequate analgesia, Colditz (1991) points out that 'there is still a deficiency of data with which to provide a definitive answer as to which treatment is best for each baby . . . a randomised controlled trial to establish whether the use of analgesia improves outcome (is) necessary'. At the time of writing this chapter, such trials are being undertaken.

In each paediatric and neonatal unit, where patients cannot speak for themselves, a proper protocol should exist for the treatment of pain, and one doctor should be responsible for its management (Boelven-van der Loo *et al.*, 1989; Andrews & Wills, 1992).

Peri- and post-surgical pain and ventilation

Pain following surgery should be anticipated and appropriate analgesics should be prescribed and given before the pain occurs (Table 6.2; Sparshott, 1989a).

Morphine is an opioid narcotic which, by binding to receptors in the CNS, alters pain perception and emotional response to pain. Its analgesic effect on the newborn is undoubted, but its action as a respiratory depressant makes it difficult to use with spontaneously breathing infants (Anand, 1993; Greely *et al.*, 1993). At one time morphine was avoided for use with the newborn because of its addictive properties, but nowadays fear of addiction has been reconsidered by both physicians and pharmacologists currently using narcotics (Anand *et al.*, 1993). Morphine is now in fact the analgesic of choice for use with newborn infants.

Morphine can be diluted in a syrup, or taken by mouth in tablet form. It can be given rectally, subcutaneously or intravenously, and this last is the route considered most suitable for fragile babies. It is invaluable for the control of pain in the mechanically ventilated infant, and should always be used in conjunction with pancuronium if the baby needs to be paralysed. Infants are more sensitive to opiates than adults; for spontaneously breathing infants, morphine can be given successfully in small bolus doses at longer intervals, or, preferably, by continuous infusion (Gauntlett, 1987). Morphine syrup is more useful in the treatment of long lasting pain, such as the mature infant with BPD who can be fed orally.

Possible side effects of morphine are: depression of respiration; seizure; hypotension; nausea and vomiting; urinary retention; and constipation. It should also be noted that preterm infants metabolise and excrete opiates more slowly than adults. Signs of withdrawal are: hypertonicity; irritability; diaphoresis; increased temperature; and vomiting. The effects of morphine can be reversed by naloxone, a narcotic antagonist.

Fentanyl and *alfentanyl* are synthetic opioids, similar in effect to morphine, which have been used in the anaesthesia of newborn infants for some time with good effect (Kay, 1973; Hansen & Hickey, 1986; Anand *et al.*, 1987). Fentanyl can also be used in combination with a relaxant in infants undergoing ET intubation, to limit the typical response of profound bradycardia and increased arterial blood pressure. A 'fentanyl–oxygen–metocurine technique' has been shown to be a safe and effective technique for preterm and ill term babies undergoing a wide variety of surgical procedures (Yaster, 1987), but withdrawal symptoms (though rare) appear to be more common with fentanyl than with morphine (Norton, 1988; Levene & Quinn, 1992). Side effects, similar to those with morphine, can be countered with naloxone.

Since symptoms of withdrawal (Neonatal Abstinence Syndrome) are frequently seen in the infant of the drug dependent mother, they must also be expected to follow a too abrupt withdrawal of analgesia in the postnatal period (Anand *et al.*, 1993; Franck & Vilardi, 1995), and in fact have been described in infants who have undergone ECMO. So far, no long-term ill effects have been seen in infants who have suffered withdrawal symptoms following analgesia given in the treatment of pain, but any neonatal pain protocol should include guidelines for the systematic weaning of infants from opioids. The flow chart in Fig. 6.4 shows how sensitive care can balance rest and quiet against the stimulation of such infants, while they are being weaned from the drug (Flandermeyer, 1995).

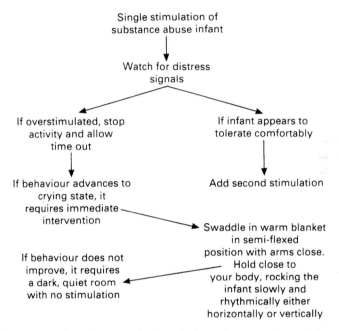

Fig. 6.4 Flow chart for stimulation of the substance abuse infant. (From Flandermeyer, 1995.)

Local anaesthetics such as *lignocaine* 1% work by blocking the triggering mechanism, and keep the nerve fixed in a resting state. Anaesthetic blocks of tender skin areas, peripheral nerves or sympathetic ganglia have the effect of diminishing the total sensory input that bombards the spinal transmission cells, and would therefore reduce the spinal output to below the critical level necessary to evoke pain. Spinal anaesthesia is effective for the repair of inguinal hernia and for lower abdominal surgery, and local anaesthetic blocks can be used for minor surgery (Aynsley-Green, 1987). Local anaesthetic used in nerve block or local infiltration of the skin can reduce the trauma of such procedures as chest drain insertion, and is thought to be safe (Yaster, 1987).

The usual dosage of lignocaine 1% used as local anaesthetic is 5 mg/kg. Excessive absorption can cause CNS depression, and there can be allergic reactions and local inflammatory and necrotic effects.

As well as immediate signs of stress, studies have shown that infants circumcised without anaesthetic later present with sleep disturbances (Emde *et al.*, 1971; Anders and Chalemian, 1974). A dorsal penile nerve block used before circumcision by Williamson and Williamson (1983) reduced infant stress, as was shown by less of a decrease in heart rate and TcPO$_2$, and less time spent crying. It would be even more humane to delay such procedures until later in infancy, when appropriate general anaesthesia can be given (Colditz, 1991).

Infiltration of a wound site with a solution of local anaesthetic can be carried out either during or after surgery; the medication most commonly used for this is *bupivacaine hydrochloride* solution up to a maximum dose of 2 mg/kg (Cornick, 1989).

For minor surgery, non-opiate analgesia such as *paracetamol* in the form of syrup (Calpol) or suppositories can be effective, either given pre- or post-operatively (Gauntlett, 1987). Paracetamol works by inhibiting the synthesis of prostaglandin at the site of the injury, so is useful for the relief of peripheral pain. It is recommended only for babies over the age of three months, but can be used for newborn infants at the discretion of a doctor and has been found both effective and safe in cases where opioid analgesia is not required. Long usage and overdose can cause liver damage, so it should not be used in the presence of jaundice. Non-steroidal anti-inflammatory drugs (NSAIDs) such as aspirin are *strongly contraindicated in newborn infants* due to difficulties in the accurate administration of small doses and possible links with Reye's syndrome (Cornick, 1989).

Pro re nata (PRN) prescriptions should be avoided in the pain management of infants, since the infants tend thereby to be undersedated (Elander, 1989).

The baby who shows by his behaviour and physiological reactions that he is coping well following surgery can be maintained in a state of well-being by sensitive nursing care (Cornick, 1989; Abajian & Sethna, 1993). He will need to be kept in a comfortable position, quiet, warm and dry. Maintenance of good hydration and, if medically feasible, early re-introduction of oral feeding will help. He will benefit from handling being kept to the minimum to begin with, and parents need to be warned of the necessity to let him rest.

Non-pharmacological pain treatment (see also Chapter 7)

There are many non-pharmacological forms of pain treatment available for adults, such as distraction, relaxation, reflexology, hypnosis, heat and cold, acupuncture, and Transcutaneous Electrical Nerve Stimulation (TENS) (McCaffery & Beebe, 1989). The well co-ordinated baby is capable of *distraction* from noxious stimuli by employing hand-to-mouth movements and non-nutritive sucking, or by returning into a lower sleep state. *Relaxation* is a learned behaviour, and as such is not available to a newborn baby as a coping strategy, but a combination of relaxation and *reflexology* can help the baby by the use of stroking and massage techniques, and by good positioning.

One form of complementary pain therapy associated with the promotion of relaxation is *Therapeutic Touch* (TT). TT can be viewed as an 'energy field interaction' which involves the use of the hands to pick up subtle cues in the patient's energy field which denote an imbalance in that field. The therapist then attempts by movements of the hands above the affected part of the patient's body, without touching, to 'clear' the field, thereby promoting relaxation (Sayre-Adams, 1994). Since TT does not involve actual physical touch, no demands are made on the patient, which could make it a suitable treatment for the relief of pain in fragile babies, but more research is needed in this area. For those interested, an accredited course for the teaching and practice of TT is available (Appendix 4).

Hypnosis has not ever been tried in the treatment of pain in babies as far as I know; although the effect of *'white noise'* (described in Chapter 7, 'Consolation by means of sound') appears to be at least part hypnotic. It is tempting to think of rocking and crooning as forms of hypnosis; I have noticed quite often that if one murmurs 'Slee-eep!' again and again in a low, rhythmical tone to an obstinate baby who is sleepy but refuses to close his eyes, after a while he will obediently do so – the problem is that the caregiver will probably do so too!

For obvious reasons it would be difficult to use *heat and cold* as pain treatment; local applications of heat or ice packs would affect the temperature of a newborn infant. The newborn infant has delicately balanced temperature control, and nothing should be done to compromise it; it is neutral temperature that will help to maintain his stability. Heat induced by gently rubbing the site of the injury may have some effect, but it may be that rubbing stimulates the nerve cells leading to 'gate control', and it is this, rather than heat, that relieves the pain.

TENS is a method of relieving pain by the stimulation of large low-threshold fibres, which raise the pain threshold by inhibiting cells which transmit injury signals. Electrodes are placed on the skin surface around the damaged area and attached to batteries which give out a series of electrical impulses, giving a tingling sensation. Its advantage is that only brief action is needed for prolonged pain relief (Melzack & Wall, 1988). As yet, no studies have shown that TENS is effective in the relief of pain in infants.

Research suggests that the ingestion of *sucrose* can be effective as an analgesic agent for newborn infants; infants who received sucrose on a dummy prior to and during circumcision were found to cry less than control infants who received water. If this is so, the combination of the self-comforting action of sucking and the analgesic agency of sucrose would seem another valuable and benign way to reduce pain and stress (Blass & Hoffmeyer, 1991).

Chapter 7
Discomfort and Consolation

Skin: the limiting membrane

The skin has both physiological and psychological functions, concerned with protection and identity; a person's well-being depends on the integrity of the skin. Since all the painful and uncomfortable procedures inflicted on a baby (as well as comfortable and pleasurable ones) concern interference with the surface of the skin, its importance as an element in physical and personality development cannot be underestimated (Sparshott, 1991a,b).

Physiological function

The skin is the house we live in; it acts as a heat regulator and a cushion for vital organs, it eliminates body waste, stores water and nutrients, detoxifies some drugs, and warns us of noxious stimuli (Wolke, 1987). The skin serves as a protective element; it must be protected itself if all these functions are to be maintained.

In the preterm infant the function of this barrier is impaired by immaturity. This occurs because:

- there are a decreased number of fibrils attaching the dermal layer to the epidermis;
- there is a thin stratum corneum layer;
- subcutaneous oedema inhibits blood flow (Lund *et al.*, 1986).

Newborn babies have an abundance of sensory fibres in the skin, which are believed to be pain receptors; as the CNS matures, so sensitivity to pain will increase. The areas of the skin most sensitive to stimuli are located in the hands and the soles of the feet, followed by the arms and legs, and finally shoulders, abdomen, chest, back and thighs. Stimulation of the hands and the soles of the feet of a bradycardic infant will provoke crying, increased heart rate and generalised body movement. Before 37 weeks' g.a. this response may be delayed or absent, but the lack of response is due to inability to modify behaviour, not inability to feel (d'Apolito, 1984).

Psychological function

The skin separates us from the dangerous world 'outside'. We talk of feelings being 'skin deep', meaning that, deep down, our identity remains untouched. We may describe ourselves as being 'soaked to the skin', but the rain gets no further than the surface. We say we are 'ruffled', or that our 'fur is rubbed up the wrong way' – all these expressions show how the integrity of the skin is connected with feelings of well-being (Sparshott, 1991b).

The integrity of the skin of a baby is part of the holding environment which he needs for development of his potential; it is also a factor in cognitive and emotional development. According to Anzieu (1974), the ego-skin (le moi-peau) is supported by three functions. In its first function, the skin is sensed as the container of all that is rich and wholesome, derived from maternal nourishment. In its second function, the skin is the boundary between 'inside' and 'outside'; it is the barrier that protects the ego from aggression coming from someone or something other than itself (protection). Lastly, in its third function, the skin is the locus and the primary means of exchange with others (communication). In the same way, Winnicott (1965) sees the skin as a limiting membrane, which lies between the infant's 'me' which is inside himself, and 'not me' which lies outside.

For most healthy newborn babies, first experiences of 'outside' are benign; this is a 'prime time', and the baby will strive to get to know the world better. The first shock of cold, noise and bright light soon gives way to warmth, nourishment and caresses – a 'stroking' of the senses. Stroking, or a warm and close contact with another person, is essential for the survival of newborn babies; those deprived of it suffer emotional deterioration (Harris, 1973). Far from stroking, the preterm and very sick baby in the NICU is subjected to a succession of aggressive procedures which might well provoke him into retreating behind a protective shell, a 'second skin', as we have discussed in Chapter 2. The stress factors shown in Fig. 2.1, experienced without remittance, may induce in the baby a feeling of helplessness in a situation where reaction, in whatever shape or form, will not save him from hurt (Sparshott, 1991b).

Discomfort

As well as the problems arising from the invasive procedures described in Chapter 6 which involve penetration of the skin surface, problems involving the skin occur from other sources:

- bruising from over-zealous squeezing of the heel during heel-prick blood sampling;
- bruising and scarring following repeated venepuncture and extravasation;
- scarring from the site of a central venous catheter;
- scarring from chest drain insertion;
- burns due to alcohol based cleaning agents, or electrodes (these burns occur through mismanagement);
- allergic reactions to adhesive strapping;
- stripping of the epidermal layer of skin beneath adhesive tape used in fixing splints and tubes, or the adhesive rings used for transcutaneous monitoring equipment.

Iatrogenic damage to the skin leading to scarring has been observed in infants two years after discharge from hospital; one child was found to have 99 scars due to needle marks (Fox, 1988). However, research has shown that nursing strategies designed to maintain skin integrity can minimise epidermal damage in VLBW infants (Gordon & Montgomery, 1996).

Choice of materials and technique

Adhesive strapping

Removal of adhesive strapping from the skin can be very painful. Tincture of benzoin has been used, amongst other products, to toughen the skin and increase adhesion, but the level of absorption through infant skin is unknown. Adhesive-removal products (although widely used) dry the skin and are readily absorbed. One way of solving this problem is to use a pectin based barrier between the skin and adhesive tape. This product moulds to the infant's skin, is not absorbed, and can be left in place for an average of $5\frac{1}{2}$ days. It can be employed for the fixing of gastric tubes, nasal prongs for low flow oxygen, temperature probes and ostomy bags (Lund *et al.*, 1986; Dollison & Beckstrand, 1995), and can help to prevent pressure in the securing of ET tubes. Pectin based barrier products are already successfully used by many NUs for these purposes.

Splinting

When splints are applied to immobilise a limb, care should be taken not to distort the limb's natural position. Many infusions are awkwardly sited, but those that occlude due to poor positioning (and not extravasation) usually indicate that the baby is battling against the splint – a sure sign of discomfort. If we imagine being immobilised for a long time in the cramped position imposed on an infant, we might think twice about how we proceed with the splinting. Many NUs use splints that are specially prepared for the newborn, which mould to the shape of the limb and which have foam tapes for non-adhesive application, but these can be expensive. Effective home-made splints can be made with flexible finger splints bent to the correct angle or with perforated splinting material which can be cut to size.

Preterm infants have diminished fat pads in their hands; skin ulcers may easily form, and care is needed to avoid pressure that could lead to skin breakdown (Anderson & Anderson, 1988). Because of the small size of the limbs, splints need to be well padded to prevent any irregularities rubbing against the skin. It is not easy to fasten a splint securely without using adhesive tape, which may cause constriction and irritation, as well as damage to the skin when removed. To avoid this, self-adhesive skin closures or porous adhesive strip can be used to secure the cannula, and strapping can be either backed over the area next to the skin, or dabbed with cotton wool to lessen adhesion. Trial of the various forms of transparent and non-allergic tapes as they appear on the market will allow nurses to decide by experience which is the most effective and the least traumatic.

Extravasation

Extravasation should not be allowed to reach such limits as to cause scarring; considerable damage can occur if i.v. sites are not closely and frequently observed for this complication, and neonatal nurses should be aware of the hyper-irritability of certain drugs. A study in 1987 showed that covering the affected area with an occlusive, hydrogel dressing can give good results in the treatment of skin damaged in this way (Rowe *et al.*, 1987). The immediate application of glyceryl trinitrate 2% ointment can also be effective. It is even better not to allow extravasation to happen, but, alas, we are all human! The use of pumps specially designed for neonatal i.v. infusion which incorporate an alarm system for line obstruction has helped to reduce these accidents.

Naso-gastric (NG) and oro-gastric (OG) tube insertion

Gastric tubes need to be firmly fixed if they are not to slip and become displaced from the stomach; removal of the fixing tape need not distress the baby unduly if gently done, or if a pectin based barrier is used. It is difficult to know whether the tube disturbs babies once in place; certainly many develop advanced skills in removing them – the tube is an enchanting thing to hold and pull! The actual insertion of the tube is accepted by individual babies in different ways; some will seem unconcerned, some will sneeze and pull faces, some will cry if the procedure is clumsily done, some will even change colour and become bradycardic. Problems from erratically placed tubes are common; a routine X-ray review of 85 tube-fed babies showed that 38 had been incorrectly placed (Weibley *et al.*, 1987); ausculating the stomach area and withdrawal of residue from the stomach will show if the tube is positioned accurately. As in all procedures, good technique comes with practice, but supervision is necessary if the beginner is not to make damaging mistakes.

Use of monitoring systems (McIntosh, 1983)

The sight and sound of monitoring systems may be initially alarming for parents, but are probably not the worst of the baby's experiences. The monitors puff, blow, pant, hiss, bubble and occasionally emit shrieks and wailing cries, but they are passive creatures – they may not 'give delight' like the sounds in *The Tempest* by William Shakespeare, but at least they 'hurt not'. Fortunately manufacturers are more aware of the importance of infant feelings than they used to be; it is possible with most modern monitoring systems to moderate alarm intensity. Monitoring must always be supported by clinical examination and visual observation; the baby must be watched as well as the monitors, and the information received from both must be compared.

Transcutaneous oxygen (TcPO$_2$) monitoring

TcPO$_2$ monitoring has proved invaluable if correctly employed, but it needs frequent calibration and false readings can be obtained in the following ways:

- Siting over the lower body may pick up right-to-left shunting through the patent ductus arteriosus.
- Siting over a bony prominence may lead to a reading that is too low.
- Air under the electrode may lead to a reading that is too high.

A combined transcutaneous sensor for measurement of both oxygen and carbon dioxide can reduce the necessity for the frequent taking of blood for blood gases. The sensitivity of the baby's skin should always be assessed before using transcutaneous sensors. The highest temperature is necessary, without risking burns, for accurate reading. The sensors can mark the skin and even cause burns if the site is not changed at regular intervals. Use of a spray-on copolymer acrylic dressing (Op-site) over the site before placing the sensor ring can reduce skin damage from this cause (Evans & Rutter, 1986). Some modern monitoring systems incorporate an alarm system whereby the caregiver is reminded to change the sensor position at pre-set times.

Pulse oximetry

Pulse oximetry supplements the combined transcutaneous sensor in the monitoring of blood gas exchange. This is a method of determining arterial oxygen saturation and pulse rate by measuring the absorption of selected wavelengths of light (Wasunna & Whitelaw, 1987). The sensor can be sited on the hand, the foot or the ankle; sometimes the calf or the forearm are used. Care must be taken when siting the sensor to ensure that the edges are not sticking into the skin. Some sensors are contained in a small clip which can be attached to a finger or toe; others have connected adhesive bands. Otherwise, some form of strapping is usually needed to secure the sensor. Strapping may impede circulation if too tight, and if too loose, movement may dislodge the sensor, leading to discomfort for the baby, and false readings from the monitor. This can be avoided if the cable is taped to the skin about 3–6 inches away from the sensor – but this involves yet more restriction of movement, and is obviously impossible for the VLBW baby.

Temperature monitors are attached by wires to thermistors on the skin, usually on the abdomen and the sole of the foot; some are disposable and are built into a flexible adhesive pad. They are non-invasive and reliable if fixed correctly, but there is a risk of displacement and consequent false readings if they are not secure, and ulceration can occur if there is undue pressure. Wires, if drawn taut, may prove an obstacle to free movement. Both central and peripheral probes need to be covered; a probe situated on the abdomen may be affected by a radiant heater, phototherapy and other environmental factors; a peripheral probe situated on the sole of the foot must be protected from convective heat loss (Mitchell, 1996). Temperature readings can also be affected by the infant's position, or a wet nappy; but it is the *trend* of the readings, rather than the actual readings, which is significant.

Apnoea monitors, which function by means of a sensor capsule adhering to the skin, have now virtually replaced the old apnoea mattresses. They are non-invasive, but if the site is not regularly changed the infant can develop an undetected skin infection beneath the sensor ring.

Electrocardiogram monitors are reliable and non-invasive. If the three electrodes do not adhere efficiently, however, (which they frequently do not in the case of the very preterm infant or the newly born infant whose skin is greasy and moist) they oblige the caregiver to disturb the baby constantly in order to replace them.

Blood pressure can be read continuously by means of a transducer attached to an arterial line, which has the added advantage of permitting blood gas estimation without the necessity for frequent invasive procedures. If a cuff is used for measuring blood pressure, restriction of the limbs can cause discomfort.

By the time this book is published monitoring systems will doubtless be even more sophisticated; new and improved models appear all the time, and manufacturers appear more baby-friendly than they used to be. In the protection of newborn babies from pain and discomfort, nurses have invented all sorts of home-made appliances and techniques, using a wide variety of materials and much imagination. Whatever works best is best, but care should be taken to ensure that material used is not potentially harmful. Here is a reminder of some dangers:

- Plaster remover can be absorbed through infant skin.
- Bands constricting the head (for fixing such things as phototherapy masks, CPAP or ET tubes, or low flow oxygen) increase the risk of intracranial haemorrhage.
- All monitoring equipment involves the use of leads, wires and tubing (the 'spaghetti junction' of the neonatal nurse's nightmare); they must neither restrict movement nor become caught about limbs, leading to obstruction of circulation.
- Monitoring equipment that is not functioning correctly causes more problems than it is worth; not only is the nurse unable to 'read' the baby's cues correctly, she is obliged to disturb him continually in order to adjust the sensors.

The proper use of appropriate equipment is important to the well-being of the infant.

Everything will be accomplished more quickly and smoothly and will be less stressful to both baby and caregiver if the correct instruments are ready to hand and functioning properly. Doctors and nurses need to be familiar with the proper usage and function of the technical equipment they employ. As each new machine arrives on the NU, so all the neonatal staff who will be handling it must learn its complexities. It is not good enough to experiment with such equipment and see what happens; burns from transcutaneous sensors, inaccurate readings, and scars from extravasation have all come about because managers failed to provide caregivers with the opportunity for proper instruction, and doctors and nurses failed to read or understand the procedural manual. This failure leads to iatrogenic trauma. If improperly used, technology will not help but inhibit the recovery of the baby.

Consolation

'Consolation', according to *Chambers Twentieth Century Dictionary*, is the 'alleviation of misery'. If it must be the role of medical and nursing staff on the NICU to inflict pain, then surely it is the role of the parents to console their own child; this is something they are capable of doing and will want to do. Parents do not always need to be taught the different ways of comforting, and they can learn from observing their baby what suits him best. This is not to say that doctors and nurses are exempt from comforting a baby; on the contrary, in the absence of the parents it is imperative that the person responsible for causing the distress should make every attempt to alleviate it afterwards. Doctors doing a round of routine blood sampling, for instance, should always take time to settle the baby and leave him comfortable, or at least arrange for someone else to do so. It is dangerous to leave a baby distressed and crying – hypoxia, bradycardia and even apnoea may result, especially in the sick preterm infant (Wolke, 1987; Brazy, 1988).

Consolation is the easiest, cheapest and most effective treatment for transitory pain; it is also undoubtedly the most agreeable for the care-giver. No-one likes to hurt a baby; to see him lying relaxed and peaceful after he has been consoled makes the infliction of pain less painful. Consolation may be given by the following means:

- massage
- stroking
- correct positioning
- music, sound and the human voice
- swaddling
- rocking
- non-nutritive sucking
- breast, cup or bottle feeding.

Tactile consolation: massage and stroking

Tactile consolation is not the same as tactile stimulation, although many of the actions are similar. Tactile stimulation consists of actions taken to attract the attention of the baby when he is alert, and is the first form of education (see Chapter 8). In consolation, the objective is to restore the baby to a state of well-being, and promote sleep.

There are many different massage techniques, which may either be used at the site of the pain or at some distance from it. Some consist of moving the skin with light repeated movements, others involve heavy pressure with stretching and pinching of ligaments, tendons and muscles. Massage helps the body to relax. It is also a process involving one person caring for another, and can instigate a feeling of security and well-being in the recipient.

Baby massage

Baby massage has been described as: 'An expression of love through a special kind of caring touching' (Auckett, 1981). Only comparatively recently has baby massage become acceptable in Europe, although it has been used for centuries in Africa, India and Latin America. In the NU, deep massage is not useful with infants as it is perceived only as another noxious stimulation. This can be seen after venepuncture, when pressure needed to stop the flow of blood frequently causes as much disturbance as the actual stab. Light rubbing or moving of the skin after a needle prick, however, often has a calming effect. Likewise, stroking the skin and very gentle containment of the limbs during a traumatic procedure can be helpful in reducing undue stress, and may help to settle the infant (Jay, 1982; Wolke, 1987).

Reflexology is the study and practice of massage of specific areas of the hands and feet which correspond to other parts of the body. It has been found that babies benefit enormously from gentle massage of these areas, adapted to the size and sensitivity of their feet: 'It is interesting to observe the pleasure and relaxation such massage can induce' (Dobbs-Zeller *et al.*, 1984).

Preterm baby stroking

Tactile stimulation in the form of stroking for preterm babies is the attempt to reproduce the tactile and vestibular stimulation the foetus receives in the womb, through contact with amniotic fluid and the wall of the uterus (White-Traut & Goldman, 1988). The preterm infant is of necessity isolated: stroking can be the means of reducing this loneliness, by way of contact with the caregiver. This contact must not be mechanical or routine, but must be made with delicacy and tenderness: 'the more sensitive the contact, the more pleasurable the sensation. It has value only when it is given and received with delight' (Huteau, 1988).

There have been many studies on the effects of tactile kinesthetic stimulation on preterm infants, giving rise to certain suppositions; these are some of the most significant:

- The most effective tactile stimulation involves pressure rather than light touch (Field, 1992).
- Very light stroking may be aversive (Scafidi *et al.*, 1986).
- Massage of chest and abdomen is aversive, possibly because these areas are associated with negative touch (Field, 1992).

- Stimulation of parts of the body, including the oral lining of the mouth, leads to an increase in vagal tone, leading to an increase in the release of insulin and other food absorption hormones, thus facilitating weight gain (Uvnas-Möberg *et al.*, 1987; Field, 1992).

Preterm infants who are overstimulated respond with changes in respiration and heart rate, apnoea, cyanosis and state changes, as we have seen. Stroking used to reduce the incidence of apnoea has had very diverse results in different studies, but this may be due to the time at which the tactile stimulation was used, and the individuality of babies. Obviously the object is to soothe the infant, not to disturb his sleep pattern. Tactile stimulation should always be dictated by the responses of the baby, and should not be continued if adverse reactions are shown.

Methods of stroking

A nursing intervention using intermittent gentle tactile contact was devised by Jay in 1982 and designed specifically for very preterm babies requiring mechanical ventilation. The method used was to warm the hands first and place them in the incubator for a time, so that they would reach an acceptable temperature. The baby's head was then cradled in the left hand without disturbing his position. The right hand was gently placed across the abdomen without touching the umbilical cord. Contact was maintained for 12 minutes, after which the hands were quietly withdrawn (containment is a modification of this manoeuvre).

TAC-TIC therapy (Touching and Caressing – Tender in Caring) designed by Adamson-Macedo consists of gentle and smooth stroking movements on the head and face, neck, upper limbs (arms, palms and fingers), torso, and lower limbs (legs, feet and toes). There are four underlying principles: gentleness, rhythm, equilibrium and continuity (Adamson-Macedo & Attree, 1994) (Appendix 4). Such a controlled involvement of the entirety of the infant's skin may well serve to restore in the infant a sense of wholeness – of the skin as a protector – lost after a sequence of invasive procedures (Sparshott, 1991b). Certainly many infants respond to TAC-TIC with every appearance of pleasure, exhibiting snuggling or preening movements whilst it is being performed; it should be discontinued if there are signs of distress.

I would add that in my experience a gentle stroking of the forehead, from the hairline to the eyebrows, or stroking forward along the top of the head, will often soothe a restless baby – much as one gentles a pony!

Physical support and position

When stress occurs, activity of the CNS causes muscle tension, an increase in heart rate, raised blood pressure and respiration – responses that intensify pain. This activity can be diminished by *relaxation*, which also reduces the muscle tension and contractions caused by pain (Howell *et al.*, 1985).

Babies relax when they are comfortable, so any action that can aid in achieving this condition will be therapeutic. The cramped environment experienced by the baby during the last weeks of intra-uterine life leads him to take up a strongly flexed position; once born, the baby is enabled by gravity to develop increasing extensor muscle activity (Turrill, 1992). Very preterm infants have not developed sufficient muscle tone to combat the force of gravity, and if allowed to lie in an extended 'frog' position will later experience difficulties in walking, crawling and sitting. The provision of boundaries which will keep the limbs symmetrically flexed, whether the baby is lying in the lateral or supine position, will help to counteract these difficulties (Fig. 7.1). Newborn babies who present an asymmetrical position (such as following a breech pre-sentation) will be more comfortable if they are initially supported in the same position until their limbs naturally right themselves.

To sustain infants in a symmetrically flexed position, boundaries can be formed by means of 'nests' or rolled soft blankets (Updike *et al.*, 1986), but these should not be allowed to impede breathing. Babies lying prone should be supported with arms close to the body, hands symme-trically up beside the head, with one hand within reach of the mouth. The hips should be raised slightly by bringing the knees up towards the chest (Turrill, 1992). Most babies appear to be comfortable in this position, but there are some who (by their subsequent movements) insist that they prefer arms and legs straight down; the caregiver can do no other than let them have their way.

Babies do not like wide open spaces; even very small babies in incu-bators will waste energy searching for a surface against which to lie. Rolled soft blankets tucked against the back or side, or giving some support to the feet, will help give a sense of security to 'range-finding' babies. For VLBW babies, fire-resistant Silicore (Spenco) mattresses, bean bags, air beds and warm water mattresses help prevent positional disorders such as flattening of the head due to immobilisation in one position. If prone-lying babies will support it, frequent changes in posi-tion should be encouraged. Sheepskins are warm and cosy, and give fingers something to grasp (not all babies like them, however, and they show this by attempting to crawl away). Small soft rolls, such as dental rolls, can be used for hands to hold, and may replace the fascination of the gastric tube.

There is no reason (except when phototherapy is required) why even the smallest baby should not be clothed. Mothers and grandmothers are ingenious at inventing soft, light garments which can be opened down

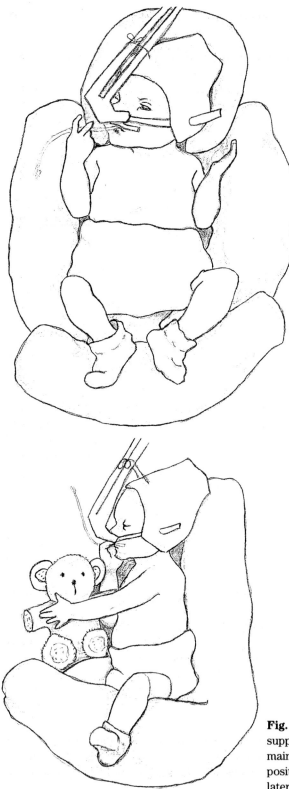

Fig. 7.1 Physical support. Boundaries to maintain the flexed position – supine and lateral.

the back, sides and sleeves, to allow for the passage of splints, tubes and wires, and to facilitate removal.

'Nests', blankets and duvets, soft garments, bonnets and boots will all help to maintain a feeling of security and comfort, besides providing warmth. Plastic bubbles help to maintain moisture and heat and allow for observation, although some babies do not find them comfortable and will try to kick them off. *Note:* caregivers should be aware that some materials are inflammable and are therefore potentially hazardous; plastic bubbles present such a hazard, and use of bean bags may add to the risk of static electricity. The dangers of the employment of all such materials should be weighed against their value in therapy.

Consolation by means of sound

Distraction enables the sufferer to diminish pain sensation by concentrating on something else, either visual or auditory. Music is sometimes used in the treatment of adult pain as a distraction technique. Those who like music can listen to favourite cassettes using a headset, and can adjust the volume as the pain intensifies or subsides (Howell *et al.*, 1985).

Babies cannot consciously distract themselves, so for the most part this form of therapy is not available to them. They are quite capable of listening, however, and there are sounds that they seem to find particularly reassuring; creatures of habit, they favour the rhythms and sounds they have become accustomed to in the womb. Intra-uterine sounds are capable of calming an infant, can stop him crying, and help him fall asleep (Murooka *et al.*, 1976).

Babies loves the sound of the human voice, and are attuned especially to the voices of their parents, to which they have become accustomed *in utero*. Cassettes of the parents' voices can be useful in calming an infant if they themselves are not present. Babies tend to have the same tastes in music as their mothers, and can recognise signature tunes of favourite radio and television programmes; on the whole, babies like soothing, rhythmical tunes.

In 1966 Wolff exposed newborn infants to a continuous monotonous sound (*white noise*) to see what effect it would have on the state of consciousness. He found that white noise has a 'powerful hypnotic and sleep-maintaining effect' on babies, except in those already vigorously crying. The baby only mildly crying, however, first stopped crying, then: 'became alert and looked around for the source of the sound; within two minutes he began to drowse, then he fell into a light sleep and finally into a regular sleep' (Wolff, 1966). Wolff did not believe that the sleep induced by white noise was entirely natural, and he suggested that artificial devices for putting a baby to sleep might not be entirely innocuous. However, as a means of soothing a distressed baby after a painful procedure, cassettes of music, parents' voices (or the gentle voice of a caregiver) and 'womb tunes' can certainly be valuable; unlike alarming monitors, these sounds *do* 'give delight and hurt not'.

Swaddling and rocking

Swaddling from birth to six months has been widely practised through the centuries – the papoose of the native American, the Italian bambino, the Baby Bunting wrapped in a rabbit skin are well known examples (Greenacre, 1953). Swaddling may reassure the infant by reproducing the sensation of being contained in the womb.

There are two aspects of restraint: the positive one of support and holding which limits but does not completely inhibit motion, and the negative, which deprives the infant of active stimulation. Babies react violently to sudden or severe restraint. If sudden severe restriction is accompanied by an angry or tense attitude on the part of the restrainer, the baby may be provoked into a strong emotional response, leading to fear and anxiety (Greenacre, 1953). Babies can be calmed by gentle restraint, however; firm and supportive swaddling which allows for some movement can be helpful in quieting the distressed baby who cannot be made comfortable by other means, such as the well baby who is not permitted oral feeds, or the baby suffering from withdrawal symptoms.

Rocking, a form of vestibular stimulation, has been shown to have a positive effect on medically stable newborn infants (Grossman & Lawhon, 1993). Albanian children who screamed when they were tightly swaddled and then bound in a cradle appeared to be calmed by rocking (Greenacre, 1953). In the NU, oscillating water beds can substitute rocking, but findings differ as to their usefulness. Water bed oscillation is said to compensate for intra-uterine floating in amniotic fluid, and is sometimes used combined with cassettes of rhythmical heart sounds. Most studies have shown benefit – a decrease in attacks of apnoea, improved weight gain, a decrease in REM sleep, fewer signs of irritability, and more frequent prolonged quiet alert states (Barnard, 1973; Kraemer & Pierpont, 1976; Als, 1986).

As far as I know, unless a water bed is used, rocking cannot be simulated in an incubator, though rocking cots are available at a price. I have seen a mechanical vibrator attached to the handles of a pram persuade a fretful convalescent baby to sleep. It is also my experience that transfer by ambulance is appreciated better by babies than by caregivers! The nicest way for babies to be rocked is in the arms of their parents.

Non-nutritive sucking/breast, cup and bottle feeding

The suck reflex is present in the foetus from the fifth month of gestation. In the newborn, it is thought to improve respiration, and thus reduce the pressure of venous return of blood to the heart. It is also believed to stimulate peristalsis and contribute to the process of digestion and elimination (Als, 1986). A well co-ordinated term baby can console or quiet himself by hand-to-mouth movements, distracting himself by sucking his fist or sucking his tongue (Brazelton, 1984). This is a highly sophisticated reaction to an unpleasant stimulus, and could be considered as a form of unconscious distraction therapy. Even small babies will suck frantically if a finger is offered to them during a traumatic procedure (Debillon, 1992). Every opportunity should be offered to the baby to console himself in this way; a preterm baby may be guided into a position with arm flexed and hand within reach of his mouth.

Non-nutritive sucking has been shown to be beneficial as a soothing mechanism. Small and sick babies must be fed by means of a gastric tube if they are not to exhaust themselves, even when they are capable of sucking. Opportunity to suck during tube feeding or the performance of a painful procedure can be provided by means of a dummy (small ones are now available), or a 'suckel' (a nipple inserted in a soft band of velvet terry cloth which the baby can hold) (Als, 1986).

If the baby is well enough, of course the best way to comfort him is for his mother to offer him the breast, or a cup or bottle feed according to the circumstances.

Consolability

Assessment of consolability is included in the NBAS. The infant's capacity for self-organisation is tested by assessing his ability to quiet himself after adverse stimulation; this is contrasted with his need for consolation from the examiner, which is offered by a graded series of procedures: facial expression; voice; hand on infant's belly; restraint of arm movements; dressing the infant; holding and rocking; and finally a dummy together with holding and rocking if all else fails – all actions designed to calm (Brazelton & Nugent, 1995). Most of these manoeuvres and the comforting actions described in this chapter are simple to perform and do not take up much time; if they are going to reduce adverse physiological reactions, then indeed ultimately time will be saved. The actions are also cheap. As to which action to take, the behaviour and physiological response of the baby will show which are the most appropriate.

Consolation should be agreeable both to the baby and the caregiver.

The 'stroking' techniques of consolation are the means by which the caregiver restores the baby's 'skin' intact; that which is broken and damaged can be restored by a loving touch – Humpty Dumpty can be put together again.

Chapter 8
Disturbance and Cherishment

The environment we should aim to create in the NU must resemble as far as possible the 'home' which would be expected to provide a healthy term baby with a cycle of day and night, nourishment, rest and stimulation, and loving attention (Sparshott, 1991c). How can we do this, while maintaining the 'safe environment' required for the fragile baby with special needs?

Day and night

Protection from light

Sleep

A regular sleep/wake cycle is established by the newborn infant over the first few months of life; the development of this cycle and the maturation of the different sleep states are seen to be closely linked to the integrity of the developing CNS (Zaiwalla & Stein, 1993). As discussed earlier, the healthy term baby can to a certain extent control his own states of consciousness, progressing smoothly from one to another. The fragile infant is not so capable, and is at the mercy of his surroundings; in the NICU, night is as the day.

That 24 hours' exposure can have a deleterious effect on the sleep cycle is certain; permanent lighting contributes to the absence of circadian rhythm, which is present in intra-uterine life (Dreyfus-Brisac, 1983). A randomised trial was undertaken in 1986 by Mann *et al.* to find out whether the physical environment (i.e. alternating night and day) has any effect, either directly or indirectly, on the subsequent behaviour of preterm infants. Results showed that infants in a day and night nursery gained weight more rapidly and slept longer than infants in a control group, suggesting that a cyclical pattern is beneficial. Curiously, the sleeping times of the babies in the day and night nursery were evenly distributed over the 24 hours, not increased at night as might have been expected; the researchers believed that this might have something to do with the influence of the hypothalamus on sleeping, appetite and weight gain.

Phototherapy

Problems arising from the use of phototherapy in the treatment of neonatal jaundice include irritation from the lights themselves, and the discomfort of exposure, since the baby must be unclothed. Plastic 'bubbles' are sometimes used to prevent heat loss from radiation and evaporation, although plastic layers of insulation, such as double-layered incubator hoods, heat shields and bubbles, will reduce the intensity of the phototherapy light that reaches the baby by as much as 40%. Complete exposure, even without a nappy, is most effective; hygiene is therefore important. Babies do not like to be naked; if the baby cannot be clothed, at least he can be provided with a rolled blanket against which to lie.

Because of the risk of retinopathy of prematurity and disturbances to the sleep pattern, the eyes of the baby under phototherapy lights must be protected. Masks can be created by using materials such as eye pads or dark covered felt; special newborn infant eye protectors are also available. No-one has yet found a way to prevent small babies displacing these masks; they are frequently to be seen wearing them over their foreheads. Probably more efficient and more comfortable for the babies (and less distressing for the parents) are specially designed orange plastic shields which can be placed across the whole head, reducing the strength of the light. An efficient and non-invasive alternative to the phototherapy lamp is the fibre optic light, or Biliblanket, which can be placed under or around the baby, leaving the eyes unaffected (Edwards, 1995).

Retinopathy of prematurity

Newborn babies, including VLBW babies whose proper environment should still be the muted darkness of the womb, are subjected to moderate-to-high light levels 24 hours a day; light levels similar to those in an NICU can cause retinal damage in animals. One study conducted by Glass *et al.* in 1985 showed a higher incidence of retinopathy of prematurity in infants under 1 kg who had been exposed to 'normal' NICU lighting, than in those who had been protected by a neutral density filter fitted over the incubator. Some of the protected babies who did develop retinopathy of prematurity were thought to have been overexposed to sunlight from nursery windows.

The following are some ways in which light levels may be reduced:

- protective window blinds which can be lowered to filter sunlight;
- night lighting or 'dimmer' lights for the whole nursery;
- individual angle-poise or spot lights by each incubator to ensure that all infants are not disturbed by emergency procedures performed on one;
- incubators covered (or partially covered) by cloth covers which protect from direct lighting but which can be folded back to increase visibility (Fig. 8.1);
- a neutral density filter or shield over the incubator;
- screens between babies receiving phototherapy and their neighbours.

In the special care nurseries with low dependency babies who do not require continuous observation, table lamps or angle-poise lamps can be used if night lighting or dimmer switches are not available.

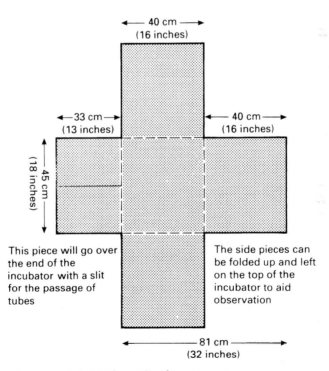

Fig. 8.1 A proposed design for an incubator cover.

Protection from noise

The foetus seems to be very sensitive to sound; the amniotic fluid which cushions the infant against mechanical shock may well amplify sound, as can be shown by the acceleration of the heart rate when a tuning fork is placed against the mother's abdomen. Studies indicate that newborn infants show a preference for sounds and voices to which they have already become accustomed *in utero*; the sound or rhythm of the mother's speech may well be recognised (Hutt, 1973: De Caspar & Fifer, 1980). In the uterus, the foetus is mainly exposed to rhythmic heart sounds and bowel sounds, but he is also accessible to muted sounds from the exterior (Saling, 1985). Some studies have suggested that the foetus is exposed to sound levels equal to those of busy city traffic, but these studies do not take into account the difference in medium between air and amniotic fluid (Henshall, 1972; Sparshott, 1995a).

British and American standards require that noise levels within the incubator should not exceed 60 dB(A), which are considered safe for an adult ear. However, noise levels do frequently exceed this level when NICU alarm systems are set off, or when ventilatory support is required (Blennow *et al.*, 1974; Bess *et al.*, 1979; Brenig, 1982; Wolke, 1987). The effect of noise on ventilated infants is hard to assess. The risk of damage to hearing from noise pollution appears to be negligible; it is generally believed that infants are not incommoded by the rhythmical, if mechanical, sound of the ventilator and the hissing of gasses, since they are already acclimatised *in utero* to sounds of 'engine tuning' and 'plumbing'. On the other hand, the behavioural and physiological responses of newborn babies to noise pollution include sleep disturbance, startles, motor arousal, and crying, a decrease of $TcPO_2$, an increase in heart and respiratory rate, and increase in intracranial pressure (Long *et al.*, 1980; Grossman & Lawhon, 1993). High frequency sounds which penetrate the incubator are mechanical, such as the slamming of incubator doors and windows, and the clap of instruments and bottles placed on the incubator top. Noise levels in excess of 60 dB(A) inside the incubator have been reached by a radio playing in the nursery, the telephone, staff talking across the incubator, and laughter in particular (Wolke, 1987).

The noise that penetrates an incubator from outside is mainly low frequency, so human voices appear muffled and indistinct, having no meaning. One consequence of a long period in an incubator is that, while the infant is unable to escape excessive clamour, the masking of meaningful noise means that he can never learn to associate a particular sound with a particular face (Wolke, 1987). Parents can be encouraged to redress this lack by talking to their babies while caressing them through open incubator doors.

How can noise pollution be reduced? Caregiver commotion and sudden sharp sounds that cause babies to startle should be avoided. The incubator can be placed away from sources of noise such as the sink, the radio and the telephone. Noise should also be a factor to be taken into consideration when choosing an incubator; a study in Sweden has shown that modifications can be made to the structure in order to limit sound. The quality of the fan, the isolation of the hood from the chassis, and modification of the portholes were some of the improvements suggested (Michaëlsson *et al.*, 1992). Manufacturers are already under an obligation to comply with British safety standards in order to reduce the noise of life support systems. If guidelines for acceptable noise levels could be set, these could be used as a standard when selecting suitable equipment for the NICU, and could encourage manufacturers to design and develop quieter equipment (Lotas, 1992).

Rest periods

When the healthy newborn baby is awakened from deep sleep he will return again to the same state; repeated awakening breaks this pattern and may provoke prolonged wakefulness. The fragile infant is even less able to support disruption of sleep:

> 'In a premature infant, active sleep and quiet sleep are poorly organised, and the respective periods of each state (wakefulness, active sleep and quiet sleep) are of shorter duration' (Dreyfus-Brisac, 1983).

Regular rest periods or 'quiet hours' can prolong sleep periods, even for fragile babies; the introduction of rest periods during the day have been seen to be beneficial, when sound and light are reduced, and nursing and medical procedures are kept to a minimum (Strauch *et al.*, 1993). 'Quiet hours' can be set aside during each eight hour shift for fragile infants, when only emergency procedures are carried out; and afternoon rest periods can be organised for all the babies on the NU.

The problem of noise pollution is one that caregivers should be able to solve, since to a large extent it is their behaviour that dictates sound levels. Neonatal staff need to be comfortable in their work, but should always be aware that shouting, loud conversation, radio playing, door slamming and careless handling of equipment is intensely disturbing to the preterm baby; the wearing of soft-soled shoes can also be encouraged. Parents, too, should understand that even if free visiting is permitted, hoards of visitors milling about at the same time in a restricted space can add to the stresses of a fragile baby. If it seems hard for neonatal staff and parents, already stressed and feeling the need to express themselves freely, to be obliged to respect periods of quiet, let it be remembered that 24 hours of loud talking, laughing and radio playing would not be tolerated in an adult Intensive Care Unit; why then should babies suffer?

Comforting sounds

There are of course sounds that will be pleasing to the baby, and that will soothe and stimulate him. Gentle speech from parents and caregivers, music boxes, recordings of the mother's voice, nursery songs and lullabies which can be played inside the incubator when he is unsettled or awake and alert, will all help the baby in his efforts to organise his behaviour.

There is evidence to show that soothing music with a flowing, lyrical melody, simple harmony, soft tone colour and easy rhythm (about 60–80 beats per minute) can promote relaxation in adults and children. A study undertaken in Vancouver showed that such music used in neonatal nurseries can help to reduce the frequency of high arousal behavioural states (stress behaviour) in newborn infants (Kaminsky & Hall, 1996).

An interesting experiment was carried out in France using a 'sound shell' cassette (*l'enveloppe sonore*) in the soothing of preterm infants. This was an attempt to use sound as a means of cracking the defensive shell in which the baby encloses himself (Chapter 2; Fig. 2.1), and to substitute a 'safety shell' (*une enveloppe sécurisante*). The idea was to calm the baby at first, and then later, when the time was right, to stimulate him (Huteau, 1988).

The team in France, with the aid of a musicotherapist, attempted to replace sounds already familiar to the foetus in the womb with the 'sound shell' cassette, which would supply the baby with low and high pitched sounds, rich in harmony. There would be a progression from deep womb sounds and music, designed to relax a stressed baby and promote natural sleep, to the high pitched sounds of everyday events at home (including the voices of parents and siblings), intended to stimulate alertness and communication.

The results of this experiment showed how different babies can be in their responses; some became agitated, cried and then settled; others listened attentively and calmly, even smiling, and seemed perfectly relaxed. One reaction that seems to confirm the doubts of Wolff as to the effect of white sound (see Chapter 7) was that certain infants were led rapidly into a state of sedation and modification of consciousness 'as if rocked in music' (Lassort *et al.*, 1988).

Temperature

Studies have demonstrated that sleep patterns can be modified by neutral temperature; certainly research has shown that disturbance of thermal regulation can lead to cardio-respiratory instability in the immature infant (Zaiwalla & Stein, 1993). Soon after birth, abdominal and axillary skin temperatures are usually close to 37°C, with a central/peripheral temperature differential of no more than 1°. The central temperature of the VLBW infant may need to be maintained at just above

37° for the differential to be within normal limits (Mitchell, 1996). If, due to cold stress, the peripheral temperature drops in the effort to maintain central temperature, the VLBW infant will waste energy in trying to make up the deficit, and the peripheral temperature may take as much as two hours to recover. Every effort should be made, then, to avoid heat loss from the incubator during care procedures (Mok *et al.*, 1991). Parents should be warned of the dangers of heat loss when they keep the incubator doors open for long periods of time; caregivers at night should watch for signs of overheating, when incubator doors are opened less frequently.

Good nursing practice will see that the baby in a cot is not affected by changes in room temperature from day to night (always possible even with thermostatically controlled heating), or by exposure to cold air during procedures. Great care is needed to see that babies moving into cots for the first time do not become too hot or too cold; one hazard the convalescent baby faces at this time is to be weighed down by a superabundance of blankets; sometimes blankets covering the baby weigh more than the baby himself!

Nourishment

Tube and cup feeding

Babies become neurologically and developmentally competent to suck and swallow at 32 weeks' g.a. (Whitworth & Topping, 1996). Even preterm infants benefit from having 'a few licks' at the mother's breast, and can be gratified by the expressing of a few drops of milk onto the nipple or directly into the mouth by hand (Lang, 1995). Many preterm babies are, however, too immature to feed themselves, even if the sucking reflex is present; these babies will benefit from NG or OG tube feeding. The baby who is too immature to breast feed can, if he is well enough, be tube fed whilst held against the breast; if he is able to suck but must remain in the incubator, he can be provided with a dummy during the feed. On this subject, opinions differ: some experts believe that babies who are to be breast fed should *not* be offered dummies, as they may become confused by the introduction of a different sucking pattern (Lang, 1995); others maintain that non-nutritive sucking during tube feeding has led to maturation of the sucking reflex, and more rapid weight gain (Bernbaum *et al.*, 1983).

A fragile baby should be fed without additional stimulation; the feeding process itself may be all he can cope with. As he improves, so quiet talking and eye-to-eye contact may be introduced (Wolke, 1987). Parents can hold their baby during tube feeding, supplying support for the trunk and shoulders, bracing his feet, and giving him something to hold (Als, 1986). If the stimulation is too much for the baby to support, he will react with 'avoidance behaviour', signs of instability connected to the attentional/interactive and the autonomic and physiological systems (Table 4.2). These will warn the caregiver to reduce the stimulation.

I have always found a satisfying way to tube feed a convalescent but still immature baby is to swaddle him and place him prone on the lap, with his head to one side. This gives the caregiver a free hand to pat and stroke his back, and to gently rock him on her knees. With this temperate stimulation, babies seem to relax while being fed. Mothers like this method of cradling while tube feeding as it means that the baby is relaxed and resting, and might not need to be returned to his incubator or cot quite so soon.

Cup feeding has proved a successful alternative method of feeding babies who are to be breast fed, but for whom a gastric tube may be inappropriate; it has the advantage of requiring little energy expenditure on the part of the baby, and since it stimulates the suck and swallow reflexes, it encourages co-ordination (Lang, 1995). Cup feeding can also be used with babies who still require gastric feeding, but who show signs of wanting to suck. If, as some believe, the two different sucking mechanisms used for breast and bottle feeding are confusing to babies, cup feeding can supply a valuable oral experience (Whitworth & Topping, 1996).

Breast and bottle feeding

If they wish to breast feed, mothers of preterm babies should be encouraged that it will be worth their while to be patient, as breast feeding can be established successfully even some weeks after the baby has been born. Meanwhile they can express their milk if the baby is too small to suck.

For the well baby, feed times are the optimal time for play, since it is then that he is most likely to be awake and alert. Whether he is breast or bottle fed, a sort of tacit conversation goes on with a baby at this time: suck – pause – jiggle of teat – suck – pause – jiggle – and so on (Bee, 1985). This is described as 'turn taking' and is one of the earliest forms of communication (Kaye, 1982). Opportunities should be provided for mothers to feed their babies in a room apart, where they can be private, quiet and relaxed. On the other hand, some mothers may prefer the company of the nursery, either for security or because they can chat with other parents.

It is a mistake to try to force a reluctant baby to feed; babies never lie, and will always have a good reason for refusal. Caregivers sometimes fall into this trap when offering a bottle to a convalescent baby who is beginning to learn sucking skills; they are so eager to succeed that they disregard the warning signals which should show them the baby is tired. Or he may be replete already, in which case he is probably being offered too much; the extra fluids required for the preterm baby will overburden the infant when he becomes more mature. In the case of the breast fed baby whose intake cannot be calculated, it is possible that breast feeding may become aversive due to the infant being forced onto the breast when he is already replete (Messer *et al.*, 1993).

Taste and smell

Newborn babies have a sense of taste and smell, as can be seen by their reactions to sweet and sour sensations (Bee, 1985). Within two weeks after birth preterm infants can identify their mother's breast milk from other milks. For the tube fed infant, cotton buds or teats dipped in mother's breast milk or the preferred formula milk will acquaint the baby with the taste; these can be offered during the time tube feeding is in progress, and a breast pad impregnated with the scent of the mother's milk can be placed near his nostrils in the incubator for him to smell. Babies can recognise their parents by mother's perfume and father's aftershave (Chaze & Ludington-Hoe, 1984). Sweet odours, therefore, can be used as a form of stimulation.

Minimal handling and stimulation

The emotional requirements of the baby requiring intensive care are very different from those of the baby preparing for home. For the 24-week g.a. baby, isolation and separation from his parents is probably not the greatest of the experienced discomforts – attention from too many different people is his problem. On the other hand, the convalescent baby, promoted from the intensive to the special care nursery, becomes isolated by default; busy staff will change and feed him routinely and are satisfied if he breathes and sleeps. If not stimulated, he is quite capable of remaining inactive all day, when it is really time he began to take some notice of his surroundings.

There is a fine line between the rest and quiet needed by the baby who is distressed by handling and the isolation experienced by the baby who is beginning to 'wake up'. To assess this moment correctly, caregivers need to concentrate on every aspect of the baby's behaviour, which is why understanding his cues is so important. All the systems we have studied for the assessment of behaviour now show their value; they can help caregivers to judge when the moment is ripe for them to free the fragile preterm infant from his isolation, and they can show when the pressure from the outside world is too much, and he needs to 'retreat' for a while.

This section concerns the way babies are 'handled' in the NU. 'Handle' is an unattractive word, but useful in this context as it can mean both a good and a bad thing; alternatives offered by *Collins Thesaurus* are 'fondle' and 'maul'. The question is: are babies in intensive and special care units 'mauled' too much or 'fondled' too little? Frequently, the answer is 'yes' to both questions.

Minimal handling

A preterm infant can easily become overstimulated. In 1983, Gorski noticed an association between the incidence of apnoea and bradycardia in infants and the 'ear-piercing cacophany of daily medical team rounds'. Using suctioning of the nasopharynx or ET tube as an example of an undesirable disturbance, Long *et al.* (1980) observed how the TcPO$_2$ of babies was affected, not only by the number of disturbances, but also by the *quality of the handling* they received. A study from Stockholm showed increases in plasma catecholamine levels in arterial blood to be most pronounced after special care nursing, which included weighing, washing the baby, nappy changing and changing the sheets in the incubator; this increase was greater after nursing care than it was after heel-prick (Lagencrantz *et al.*, 1986). Crying, supine positioning, over-handling, noise, lack of opportunity for non-nutritive sucking, and *badly organised timing* for medical and nursing procedures, can all have an adverse effect on the arterial oxygen saturation of the preterm infant, especially the infant suffering from respiratory distress (Als, 1986).

Preterm infants are handled on average about 130 times in 24 hours, with the total time occupied by handling about 3.7 to 4.3 hours during the 24 hour period (Wolke, 1987). Main sources of disturbance are the nursing and support staff, then the paediatricians, and lastly the parents (Korones, 1976; Murdoch & Darlow, 1984). It is the most fragile infants that are handled the most frequently. If a baby is so ill that he requires continuous monitoring and the undivided attention of one nurse, then some way has to be discovered to provide him with the opportunity to rest. Care should be grouped to ensure the baby long periods of undisturbed quiet. This includes basic nursing care and such interventions as blood-taking, X-rays, physical examination, ultrasound and chest physiotherapy (Lawhon, 1986). Routines that are known to have an adverse effect, such as weighing and suctioning, can be reduced to the minimum necessary for safety.

Grouping care requires collaboration between all caregivers, including parents. Nurse, doctor and parents can consult with each other on the most convenient time for routine procedures. However, one of the problems with minimal handling and grouping care is that babies can be relatively ignored between interventions (Lawhon, 1986). If the baby shows signs of stress he must be comforted; restlessness and crying should not be allowed to continue. The 'Kangaroo' method of placing the preterm ventilated baby between the mother's breasts against her bare skin (or for that matter against the father's chest) has been shown to be beneficial to both, but should not be continued if behavioural and phy-siological cues show the baby to become stressed. If the ventilated baby is sufficiently stable, however, Kangaroo holding is of great benefit in the formation of attachment (Whitelaw, 1986; Gale *et al.*, 1993; Affonso *et al.*, 1993; Blackburn & VandenBerg, 1995). While out of the incubator and cuddled by the parents the baby should be protected from bright lights and loud noise, which can distract and disrupt parent and infant inter-action.

The way parents handle and care for their high-risk infants is now believed to influence later neurological functions such as learning and language. Parents are frequently intuitive in their handling of their babies (Wolke, 1987); their movements are gentle and benign, beginning with stroking of the back and limbs, accompanied by talking, sometimes just touching the baby's hand with a finger. Unfortunately, in the case of the stressed, very preterm or fragile baby, even this gentle contact can interfere with an infant's rest. Faced with a limp and unresponsive baby, parents will make great efforts to get him to respond to them, but a study conducted by Field in 1982 showed that the more the mothers of high risk babies insisted on attempting face-to-face interaction, the less the infants were likely to respond. If a mother was asked to decrease her persistence and simply copy her baby's movements, taking her cues from him, this would produce a striking increase in the infant's gaze.

What actions can be taken to console and comfort the fragile infant, if stimulation does not benefit him? The technique of containment can be attempted, as described in Chapter 6. If even this proves too over-whelming, the best activity is non-activity; and it is important to establish a minimal handling protocol, which all caregivers should respect (Table 8.1). The baby in need of minimal handling and maximum quiet should be nursed in the part of the NICU that is furthest away from such disturbances as sinks, telephones and the main door where people are continually coming and going. Parents, too, can be made aware of the disturbance caused by too many visitors, and can make their own restrictions.

Stimulation

If over-stimulation is harmful to the very ill or very immature baby,

Table 8.1 Minimal handling protocol.

Protect from light
Darken incubator, crib
Place blanket over end of table bed
Shade infant's eyes when handling

Protect from noise
Remove phones; lower loud speakers, radios
Pad all trash receptacles
Pad noisy doors
Give shift report away from bedside
Close incubator doors quietly

Caregiving
Allow 2–3 hour periods of undisturbed rest
Cluster nursing care activities. (Be careful not to rush or be abrupt. Work efficiently with
    gentle handling. If still stressful for infant, try to allow short rest period between each
    activity)
Do not do routine postural drainage (PRN only)
Do not do routine suctioning (PRN only)
Use two-person suctioning if possible

Postioning
Position prone or side-lying
Cover/wrap/swaddle
Use blanket rolls to tuck around sides/back/feet/head
Provide suck and grasp opportunities

(From VandenBerg, 1995.)

stimulation at the right time is essential for the healthy one. Tactile
contact is the infant's first form of giving and receiving communication,
and depriving him of this may compromise his future development.

As discussed in Chapter 1, learning theorists maintain that observation
and learning of the environment come about as a result of reinforced
practice. Since it is likely that the preterm infant is born at a time when
maximum brain growth is occurring, it is evident that appropriate
stimulation will be necessary for the successful development of early
skills (Rushton, 1986). The baby is born with certain reflexes, such as
rooting, sucking and hand grasp, but all these abilities have to be
practised. A sound, such as the mother's voice, needs to be associated
with something seen, such as her face, so that all the mechanisms of
memory, recall and recognition can be set in motion.

The NICU must therefore provide opportunities for learning; but
opportunities for learning in an incubator are limited, as faces are the
wrong distance away and voices are muffled and distorted. Most of the
actions of consolation already described in Chapter 7 can be used, in a
different context, to stimulate. Stimulation of the senses can begin gently
with the preterm baby, and can then progress as the child 'convalesces'

until he is ready to go home; an example of an infant stimulation care plan involving all the senses is given in Appendix 3 (Chaze & Ludington-Hoe, 1984). Stimulation is most effective when the baby is in an awake and alert state, which he shows by lying quietly, eyes open, looking around him, perhaps turning his head to a voice. He will then be receptive to a provocative or 'interesting' environment (Wolff, 1966) (Fig. 8.2). The baby who wishes to be 'left alone' will appear limp and floppy, refusing to engage in eye contact (Fig. 8.3).

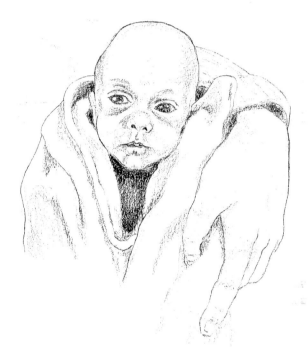

Fig. 8.2   This baby is ready to be stimulated. (From Sparshott, 1989c.)

Touch: stroking and massage – preterm infants

Obviously caregivers must learn from their observations of individual behaviour what methods of stroking are best suited to the preterm baby; by trial and error, they can learn what actions will best lead to relaxation and stabilisation, and which points of contact the infant is likely to reject. As to the form of massage, the following has been recommended by Field (1992) for use with fragile babies:

(1)   Take very slow strokes (approximately 10 per minute) from top of head down to nape of neck, and then back up again.

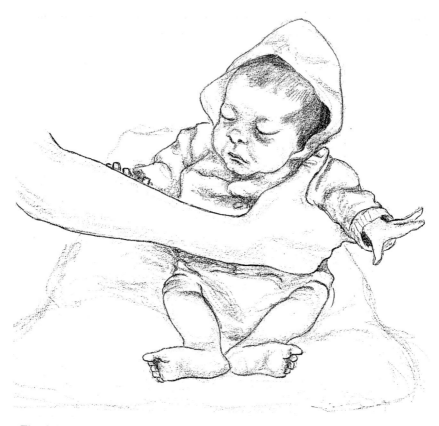

Fig. 8.3 This baby wants to be left alone. (From Sparshott, 1989c.)

(2) Then stroke shoulder region, back region, and down and up arms and legs – this massage lasts 5 minutes in prone position.
(3) With infant in supine position, apply 5 minutes' extension and flexion of upper and lower limbs (avoid chest and stomach).
(4) After this, repeat massage with baby lying on his stomach.

Tactile stimulation of this nature can be of benefit to a preterm baby in an incubator, deprived of the supreme contact of being held in the arms of his parents, but of course it should be discontinued if the infant shows signs of distress (Field, 1992). The need for individual assessment should be emphasised; stimulation needs to be carefully timed so as not to interfere with rest periods, and adverse reactions on the part of the baby should warn the caregiver when to stop (White-Traut & Goldman, 1988).

Massage – term babies

The act of massage gives pleasure to most infants. When such stimulation is used, parents should certainly participate, since it is their touch the baby must learn to recognise. Auckett suggests that:

'Massage should flow from top to toe, starting with the head and following on to face, neck, shoulders, arms, chest, belly, legs and feet. Then, turning the baby onto his belly, head, neck, back, buttocks, legs and feet. Finish with long, sweeping strokes from head to toe.'

The mother should keep her nails short, or use only the balls of her fingers (Auckett, 1981).

Bath times are good times for tactile stimulation; the mother can exercise her baby's limbs and play with him, and while he is naked, hold him against her bare skin. Baby massage for the well baby using organic and essential oils has been described by Walker in both book and video (Appendix 4); this massage is designed to improve co-ordination and posture, and promote flexibility and mobility. Passive extension of the arms and legs is also beneficial; babies do not like to straighten their limbs, but skilful massage can persuade them to do this willingly (Walker, 1995).

Sound stimulation: voice and music

Mothers have crooned and sung lullabies to their babies for thousands of years. As she talks or sings to him, the mother plays a game with her baby using phrases with pauses in between. It is the *harmony* of the sound and its *repetition* that is important if she is to hold his attention. The 'baby' voice is not to be despised – the cooing, singing quality of the voice, which is repetitive by instinct, will frequently evoke an intense concentration from the infant in an alert state, as is shown by his fixed gaze, his stillness and the way he holds his head. Baby talk should be alternated with adult speech, but this will happen naturally if both parents are present.

The same gentle, reassuring tone of voice can be used to gain the attention of a preterm baby in an incubator. The parent whose baby is grasping her/his finger and who sees that his eyes are open should certainly talk to him, repeating his name, and the response will show when he is happy to listen. If the sound stimulation is too much for him, he will close his eyes and relinquish his grasp, maybe fidget and extend his fingers, as though he wishes to push the sound away. This wish should be respected.

In the absence of the parents, cassettes of their voices can be used to attract the attention of the infant when he is alert. Parents should repeat the baby's name frequently, speak slowly and include some baby talk (Chaze & Ludington-Hoe, 1984). Caregivers, too, in the absence of the parents, can talk and sing to the babies at times of optimal attention – anyone is capable of singing to babies!

Sounds of heart beat, and musical toys and boxes are also valuable sources of stimulation – a music box played regularly when a baby is settled after feeding can give great pleasure, as is seen by the relaxed position of the body, eyes turned attentively towards the sound.

Vision

The newborn infant lacks sharpness of vision; he cannot focus on an object. It appears that babies for the first 6 to 8 weeks of life spend their time searching *where* objects are; they look for the edges of things rather than individual features (Bee, 1985). The exception seems to be the human face. Babies will concentrate on places of sharp contrast, such as eyes and mouth, but they can tell the difference between the photograph of a real face and one that has been scrambled (Goren *et al.*, 1975). Babies only a few days old can recognise enough to be able to copy expressions, and even commit them to memory.

The newborn baby sees best at about 25 to 40 cms (Atkinson & Braddick, 1982). From this distance, the caregiver can make face-to-face contact with the baby, looking into his eyes, and talking to him at the same time to provide the movement that he may need to hold his attention. When he has had enough, he will become restless or inert, and his eyes will wander. The preterm baby will only be able to support eye-to-eye contact for a very short time.

As babies grow older, so their vision becomes more acute. They appear to prefer shapes with curves and large designs. Some investigators believe that black and white are the preferred colours, and provide sheets and cards with black and white pictures of faces which can be placed at eye level when the infant is lying prone (Chaze & Ludington-Hoe, 1984). Others suggest that the medium colours of yellow, green and pink are preferred to the stronger colours of red, orange and blue. Some babies seem to like the sight of their own faces in a mirror; of course, they cannot recognise what they see, but perhaps it is the roundness and the soft colour, and the movement, which they find pleasing. Whichever or whatever it is, the attention the infant pays to the stimulation will show whether or not he likes it.

Soft toys in incubators, and cards or books with bold designs, provide stimulation for the preterm infant, but these should be placed where he can see them when he is alert, and removed from view when he is tired or stressed. For the older baby, mobiles can be attractive, especially those which revolve and play a tune at the same time. They must, however, be placed at a distance where the baby can see them. The most successful stimulation of all is the mobile face of mother or father, smiling at their child. It seems that the face of the father has a particular attraction, particularly if he has a beard – maybe because of the strong curves.

Motion: cuddling and rocking

In countries such as India and Africa, the baby is often carried in a sling against the body of the mother while she works; carried against her in this way, the baby enters into an intimate relationship with his mother, which stimulates him at the same time. He moves and bends when she does, follows her rhythm, participates in all her activities, and feels her emotions. This close contact calms and stabilises him, renders his body more supple, reinforces his muscle tone, will help him to sleep and at the same time give him a sense of well-being (Maury, 1988). It is a perfect introduction to the outside world.

The preterm infant is deprived of all this; nor is there any way that maternal contact can be supplied if the baby is too ill to be cuddled. The Kangaroo method of holding the baby naked between the mother's breasts cannot be practised if he is too fragile. As already described, comfortable positioning and the undemanding action of containment may be tried for their effect.

The convalescent newborn baby also tends to miss out on cuddles if the parents are not available. Nurses are often overworked, and the baby will do well to be changed, fed and replaced in his cot without more ado, but the well baby needs the stimulation of motion. Many babies enjoy being carried about the ward after feeds, either in the arms or over the shoulder where they can see what is going on. Sometimes time can be saved this way, since it is an excellent method of aiding the baby to bring up wind, and will dispose him to sleep afterwards. A Kangaroo type of baby carrier or baby sling can be used to transport a baby around with the caregiver (Auckett, 1981; Cunningham *et al.*, 1987), and is particularly useful for the baby who has been a long time in hospital; used by the mother, it will help promote mother–infant relationship. A rocking chair in the nursery or breast feeding room can be provided for mothers to rock their babies while they are feeding them.

Other methods of promoting and prolonging an awake state are the use of hammocks or baby chairs, where the infant may sit fairly upright, with a mobile at hand to look at or coloured balls on a string to play with.

Perhaps the best illustration of the ill effects of failing to provide an appropriate environment is the following story told by Monique Huteau, at that time nursing superintendent of a premature baby unit in France.

The effect deprivation of the appropriate stimulation can have on an infant was observed by the neonatal team of a premature baby unit in

Poitiers, who were experimenting with the *sound shell* cassette. Emanuelle, born at 26 weeks' g.a. and weighing 960 g, was very ill at the beginning and remained in intensive care on life support machinery for seven weeks. After this she was transferred to the Premature Baby Unit. Two days after her arrival, she was introduced to the sound shell cassette. At first agitated by this, after five days she would open her eyes, lift her arms, and turn her head towards the sound. She could calm herself, relax and smile at the sound of the cassette.

Three weeks later, however, she began to give rise to anxiety. She became cyanosed and bradycardic during feeds, refused eye contact, became irritable and cried frequently. No medical reasons were found for this, and eventually the team came to the conclusion that, because of changes in staff and an excessive work load, Emanuelle had become a little neglected; the cassettes had only occasionally been played. The staff reconsidered their attitude towards Emanuelle. The cassette was played every day at the same time, morning and evening. The baby was caressed and cuddled by the staff, who even allowed her to participate in the activities of the unit in a carry-cot, or held against the body of the caregiver in a Kangaroo carrier. Emanuelle regained her state of well-being, engaged in eye contact, was interested in all about her, and became increasingly alert.

Monique Huteau makes the following wise observation: 'Through this painful case, we realised how much a baby needs to be surrounded, loved, stimulated all the time by those who care for her. We could see the danger of bringing an infant to a certain height of performance, then brutally diminishing this solicitude. The baby has the sensation of being abandoned, and will tend to regress in consequence' (Huteau, 1988).

Part III
The Holding Environment

Chapter 9
Caring for the Family

(The quotations are taken from an article written by Béatrice Berger, a young French mother whose baby was born at five and a half months' g.a. (Berger, 1981))

'Chloé was born that sad morning, and I was totally unprepared for all that was going to happen.'

Neonatal intensive care is disturbing to parents; most of them hate the frenetic atmosphere created by stressed staff coping with a high work load, and are worried by the constant noise and bustle. The apparatus of 'high technology' does not go well with newborn babies, whom one imagines lying in comfortable cots, surrounded by toys and pictures and admiring relatives, in a cheerful room decorated with nursery wallpaper. This is a far cry from incubators, monitors, wires and tubes. Something is needed to reassure parents that their babies are growing individuals, not objects in a factory being put together on a production line.

The Neonatal Unit

'From the first, we were encouraged to visit the unit as often as possible, to caress Chloé, to talk to her, and above all not to forget that she was alive and had need of our love.' (Béatrice)

First impressions are important, and the entrance to the department should be welcoming. If a preterm delivery is likely, it will help parents to have some idea of what an NU looks like, and visits before the baby is born will help to prepare them if later on their baby needs to be admitted. It is a good idea at this point to show parents 'before and after' photographs of babies, so that they can see for themselves that premature delivery can have a successful outcome.

A booklet describing the unit can be made available to the parents of babies who are admitted, and should include a ground plan of the unit, descriptions of the roles of the neonatal staff, and all other relevant information, such as arrangements for visiting, where they can obtain refreshments, and to whom they should refer for special needs. A booklet giving information on prematurity may also be helpful to the parents of preterm babies, such as Moore's *Born Too Early* (1995), which includes illustrations and descriptions of equipment used.

The Neonatal Unit team

'The doctors and nurses were very humane and attentive, as much to the feelings of the babies as to the anguish of the parents.' (Béatrice)

First encounters with the neonatal staff are of paramount importance. Parents like to know to whom they are speaking; members of staff can wear badges with their name and function, and a board can be set up in a prominent place with photograph, name and function within the team of everyone the parents are likely to meet. Nowadays, doctors need not wear white coats but can remain in civilian dress, which helps to make the atmosphere less formal. Nurses wear a uniform, but the heat of the nurseries gives an opportunity for this to be casual and comfortable. Christian names are usually acceptable between parents and staff, especially in the case of parents whose baby is in hospital a long time – but this should not be taken for granted; it is tactful to find out first how parents want to be addressed.

A 'named nurse' is usually allotted to each baby on admission, which gives the parents a definite person to whom they can refer in trouble. The nursing skill-mix on most NUs may make this difficult to maintain when the baby graduates from intensive to special care, and is likely to be cared for by different staff who must become attuned to his changing needs. It will, however, help parents (and babies) if there can be some continuity in the nurses providing individual care, since they are likely to feel more relaxed and secure with someone they know; continuity of care will also help nurses to establish a warm relationship with a family, even in situations that are particularly stressful. Many a neonatal nurse feels impelled to continue caring for a critically ill patient and his deeply distressed parents in spite of heartache; there is a feeling of 'seeing it through' together, which is comforting to parents, who feel that the nurse cares about them.

Parents must be able to trust the neonatal staff, and this means that they must feel free to ask questions and expect to receive honest answers. Policy must be decided on how and by whom such replies are given. The tendency is for parents to ask questions of everyone concerned with their baby, particularly if he is very ill. This is often considered to be 'playing off' the staff against each other, but it does not necessarily mean that the parents distrust the person they listen to the first time; frequently they will block what they hear from their memory, particularly if the news is not good – or if it is good but they dare not believe it. It is sometimes difficult for neonatal staff to know how to reply to direct questions, particularly if a diagnosis is not confirmed, since the voicing of suspicions may worry the parents for no reason. If the answer to a question is 'I don't know' it is best to say so, even though parents usually find this answer difficult to accept and will press for more. However, since most of the time the outcome will be good it is wisest to be optimistic; parents will feel more free to relate to a baby in whose future they can believe (Brewin with Sparshott, 1996).

Parents want to talk and to be heard. The doctor who is discussing the progress of a baby will give more pleasure to the parents if it is indeed a discussion, not a lecture in biochemistry. Nurses, too, should be careful not to reduce the parents' already insecure confidence by emphasising their own technical skill and efficiency; explanations should be made in simple language, without jargon.

Nursing care of the parents is indeed invaluable at this stage; they will welcome support and encouragement, provided the nurse is not tempted to treat them as children themselves. Parents are quick to recognise patronage. The sooner parents can be shown that they are necessary to their baby's well-being, the sooner they will be able to recognise him as their own.

The family

'The family' can either be considered as the nuclear family consisting of parents and siblings, or the extended family which includes grand-parents and other relatives (Morris, 1994). Free visiting for the parents of babies in the NU is now commonly accepted, but other visitors should only come accompanied by the parents, until the staff are familiar with those trusted family members whom the parents wish to be allowed to visit freely. Nor should it be taken for granted that grandparents, aunts and uncles are automatically going to be welcome to the parents. NU staff will need to be cautious and tactful until the individual family set-up is understood.

Nowadays family relationships tend to be complex; the mother's partner may well not be the father of the baby, the mother herself may be very young and dependent on her own parents; conflicting interests are only too frequent. If the mother so wishes, her present partner will need to be accepted as the future 'parent', especially as the baby may be taking his name. Sometimes, however, it may be her mother or even a close friend who gives her the most support; she will need the com-passionate support of others outside the NU team, and if she is alone she should be encouraged to find someone she trusts to help her share her worries. It is sad for a young girl to try to cope alone with all the stresses of a preterm birth or a sick baby. Social workers can always be contacted in cases of need, if the mother agrees, and in some cases the social worker may be the person to whom she feels she can best turn for help and understanding. All these points will have to be made clear before discussions are held and decisions made as to the baby's future.

The parents

When parents first visit the intensive care nursery, staff concentrating on the baby may be tempted to explain in detail the functions of the monitors and ventilators to a couple who would prefer to know how their baby is feeling, if he is hurting, if all his limbs are where they should be, and what is going to happen to him. The nurse at this point may not be able to give answers to all these questions, but she can show the baby to his parents, refer to him by gender, ask if he has a name, and reassure them of his present well-being as well as she is able. Explanations of equipment used can come later.

That the baby may feel discomfort should not be denied; parents can see this for themselves. But even at this early stage it is not too soon to explain to parents that much may be done to make their baby comfortable, and that in achieving this they themselves are indispensable. Parents would rather hear what a little fighter their baby is in his struggle for survival, than be told that he feels nothing when it is plain that he does: 'Some nurses did not understand why small things, such as the pain caused by removal of plasters, should cause parents so much distress when the babies were in a critical state,' one father said. 'To us, any way in which we could alleviate Bethany's pain was worthwhile, on the basis that everything helped' (Hughes & Hughes, 1993).

'Parents', then, in this context, may be taken to mean mother and father/partner; the persons whose responsibility the baby is going to be. Parents are individuals who may have different needs; however, many anxieties are common to both, and in decision-making it is best if both parents are consulted together; they can give each other mutual support.

The mother

Caplan and colleagues (1965) held that the mother of a preterm infant needs the following abilities:

- to understand the problem realistically (a *cognitive* coping mechanism);

- to understand her own feelings and express them verbally (an *effective* coping mechanism);
- to ask for help (a *social* coping mechanism).

If the right environment is provided for the infant in intensive care he is not likely to suffer in the long term from early separation from his mother; it is the mother's separation from him that causes so many problems. It may be that damage to the relationship between mother and baby comes about because she is *prevented* from having access to him rather than lack of contact itself. She may be daunted by the environment of the NU, and resent the restraints on spontaneous interaction. But given the right environment, parents, like their babies, have immense powers of recuperation and adaptation.

At one time it was believed that 'bonding' from birth was essential for the physical and emotional development of the infant, but this belief has been modified. In fact the idea of attachment as a sort of 'magical glue' can cause considerable distress to parents who feel that their failure to bond in the first days will have life-long consequences (Gaussen & Hubley, 1987). It is now believed that the complex process of attachment between infant and caregiver takes place over a long period of time. Separation during these earlier days, though distressing to parents, will not prevent the relationship between them developing normally once they are all reunited. This concept, explained to parents, may help to alleviate the guilt and anxiety they feel. The extent to which the mother believes separation to be important may be a significant factor in later development; encouraging a positive attitude towards her fragile infant is imperative.

Just as the preterm infant is expelled from the womb before he is ready to leave it, so the mother experiences the premature expulsion of her baby as a mutilation; 'It was as if they ripped a piece of my guts out,' was one mother's description of her feelings (Cramer, 1976). The baby is born before the mother's love has ripened; her love is as immature as he is. She may well feel resentment towards the baby whom she is unable to help, but whose sufferings she sees as the cause of her own distress.

Together with other complex emotions, the mother of the preterm baby goes through a process of mourning. She feels:

- Disbelief   'This can't have happened to me!' She does not perceive her preterm baby as 'real'.

- Anger   'Why has this happened to me?' She is angry at the events (often unidentified) that have brought this violation upon her. This anger may be directed at her partner, the baby, the neonatal staff, but basically it is undirected; she is angry with Fate.

- Guilt   'It must be my fault.' She can feel guilty for almost any reason and for no reason.
- Inertia   'There's nothing I can do about it.' Listlessness and apathy are the result of shock and revulsion. She is helpless in the face of events she cannot control and a baby whose needs she does not understand.
- Grief   'I dare not love this baby.' The mother not only grieves for the baby she dreamed of during her pregnancy, but must also face the possibility of losing the fragile being to whom she has in fact given birth.
- Acceptance   'After all, this is my baby; I love him, and must do my best for him.' She accepts that her dream baby never existed, and turns towards loving the 'changeling' that now in her perception comes into being as her own flesh and blood (Sparshott, 1993).

These are all powerful emotions; let us now examine them, and see how the mother can be helped to overcome the first five, and arrive safely at the last.

Disbelief

'I understood nothing, the reality was too sudden and too hard.' (Béatrice)

Behind every fantasy of the beautiful chubby dream-child lurks the spectre of malformation and deformity – the baby who is not 'normal' (Richards, 1978). If her baby is taken away from her, the mother will believe the very worst; her imagination may turn her preterm baby into a grotesque monster, until she has seen him. She should be provided as soon as possible with a photograph, so that at least she can see for herself that her baby is 'all in one piece'.

When she does see him for the first time, the mother may still, if the baby is very small and fragile, be intimidated and even revolted by his appearance. It is no use telling her he is beautiful – that is not how he appears in her eyes. Neonatal staff should remember that they are accustomed to seeing very immature-looking babies; to parents it is a great shock. The nurse can take a positive approach, pointing out such details as the tiny nails, the miraculous nature of fragile hands that can grip a finger with such strength. It may help parents if they can perceive their baby as being entirely normal – only normally they would not be in a position to see him at this time! Eventually, he will grow into proper baby-shape. In the meantime, the visual shock may be eased by seeing a 'rogues' gallery' of photographs, with pictures of other babies as small as their own, and how they appear as children later on.

A new mother usually likes to talk to others who have babies already on the unit; looking at babies who are at different stages of development and talking to their parents will help her to envisage the possibility that her own baby may grow. It is comforting for mothers to know that others have survived the same ordeal. Some have written little books about their experiences which are kept in the NU for all to read.

It is important for the mother to feel that she can herself take part in creating a temporary 'home' for her baby in the NU which will best help him to thrive. In this she may be encouraged by the booklet written especially for the parents of preterm infants: *This is Your Baby: How to understand your baby and what to do to help him grow* (Sparshott, 1989c). The booklet explains very simply how preterm babies develop, why they behave the way they do, how to understand their behaviour, and how they are likely to respond to different forms of comforting. Contained in the booklet are tables showing signs of stress and well-being, ways to soothe and comfort, and methods of stimulation when the baby is ready (Table 9.1.)

Table 9.1 Signs of stress and well-being.

Signs of stress
Crying
Grimacing, making faces
Eyes squeezed tightly closed
Coughing, sneezing and yawning
Hiccoughing, gagging or being sick
Fingers splayed – hand appears 'star shaped'
Tremors, startles, twitches
Either extreme limpness, flaccidity
    or frantic activity, violent movements of limbs
Very uneven breathing, pauses in respiration
Colour changes (becomes pale, mottled, grey or blue)

Ways to soothe and comfort your baby
Talk to him in a gentle voice
Stroke his body or his limbs
Gently stroke his forerhead
'Contain' his head and body in your hands[1]
Hold his hand – let him grasp your finger
After he has been disturbed, place him in his preferred position
Tuck him or cuddle him into his blanket
Cuddle him, holding him close to you with his head supported (not with his chin on his
    chest!)
Hold him to nestle against your shoulder
Rock him in your arms
Give him something to suck (if he can do so)
Bring him a cassette of your own voice to comfort him when you are not able to be there

Table 9.1   Continued.

Signs of a state of well-being
A relaxed and comfortable position
Peaceful sleep – no rapid eye movement
Eyes open and intent, alert appearance
Head and eyes turn towards sound of voice
Movements smooth, not jerky
Hand will clasp a finger
Hand relaxed with fingers folded
'Preening' movement of body when stroked
Movement of hand to mouth
Sucking or rooting movement
A good, even colour of skin
Breathing is even, not laboured

Ways to stimulate your baby (when he is ready)
Talk to him, while looking into his face from about 10 inches away
Stroke him[2]
Sing to him
Bring him small soft toys he can grasp
Bring him little books or pictures with brightly coloured designs for his cot
Bring him a lullaby music box to play after his feeds, before he goes to sleep
Bring him cassettes of restful music
Play with him at bath times, stretching and massaging his limbs[3]
Older babies enjoy looking at mobiles

---

[1] If your baby seems stressed and anxious, but is very small and fragile, you can give him comfort without stimulating him. Without moving your baby, gently cup your hand over the top and back of his head. Then place your other hand lightly over his trunk, so that you are 'holding' him without stimulating him. By doing this, you are giving your baby the comfort of your presence without asking him to give anything in return.
[2] 'Stroking' is done by sliding the fingers lightly along the surface of the skin.
[3] 'Massaging' is done by using the fingers to move the muscles beneath the skin. To begin with, use the lightest 'feather' touch until you see how he likes it. Massage from top to toe, and don't forget to include both arms and both legs, so that your baby doesn't feel unbalanced! If you have long fingernails and don't want to cut them, make sure you only use the balls of your fingers or the palms of your hands. (From Sparshott 1989c.)

If the mother can understand that the limitations of her infant's responses are due to him being too immature to cope with the world outside, she will help to protect him from over-stimulation, and learn from his cues when he wants to be touched and when he wants to be left in peace. It can be explained that to expect interaction from him at this stage is rather like asking a child of four to behave like a boy of fourteen! Instead of protecting him inside her body, she can be shown how to give him comfort outside her body, by using the technique of containment, or one of the other consolatory techniques already discussed in Chapter 7.

One of the greatest disappointments for the mother (and probably the most frustrating) is her inability at first to put her preterm baby to the breast, but if she wishes to breast feed she can be reassured from her first visit of the importance her milk will have for him. Later, she will be shown how to express her milk, and she should see the milk offered to her baby with her own eyes. When she has enough confidence, and when he is well enough, she herself can offer him a taste of her milk on a cotton bud; the sight of her tiny baby sucking is encouraging to a mother deprived of the intimacy of breast feeding. Some mothers like to place a used breast pad in the incubator, thus stimulating the olfactory system of their preterm infant. If the mother wishes to give her baby formula milk, this is something which can be established from the beginning and should not be made a subject of guilt. Later on, tube feeding is also a technique that can be taught to parents, and as soon as they feel confident they can give the baby tube and bottle feeds.

Anger

'My first reaction was anger, I did not want to see this tiny foetus ... I became known as the "nuisance" of the unit because I sometimes commented on things that revolted me ...' (Béatrice)

Anger can be a destructive emotion, especially if it is directed at an imaginary source. Neonatal staff will need great patience with angry parents, particularly as they frequently seem to be searching for something to criticise or someone to blame. Distraught parents in their anger can say hurtful things that are hard to forget. Unfortunately, it is only too easy for staff to resent an angry parent, whom they consider ungrateful and unjust, and this resentment may persist long after the parent has 'simmered down'.

Anger and insult have to be tolerated and forgotten, even if that is hard for doctors and nurses who are doing their best for the baby; responding to abuse with anger may give feelings of temporary relief, but this is self-defeating in the long term. Sometimes it may help to encourage the parents to talk about their anger, and give it a name – frustration perhaps at their lost hopes and the disruption of their lives. The parent of the sick or preterm baby should be heeded with compassion, attentively and without argument. Then, when all feelings are out in the open, it might be possible to turn all that wasted energy into a more profitable direction. This should not be done by justifying the actions of the neonatal staff, but by suggesting how the parents can themselves help their baby. Parents are understandably angry when they see their child traumatised; they have every right to be so, even if fundamentally they know that it is for his ultimate benefit. It can be suggested to them that if they are the ones to comfort and console, that is how their hands will come to be recognised by the baby (Brewin with Sparshott, 1996).

Guilt

> 'I didn't dare telephone because I had come to believe my anxiety was more my own imagination than reality ... I ended up not daring any more to speak of my fears.' (Béatrice)

The mother of the preterm baby is overwhelmed by feelings of guilt at what she perceives to be her own failure. She may seek for an imagined defect in her person and personality; she has received a brutal blow to her pride (Cramer, 1976). The emotional problems of the mother who gives birth to a baby before term have been described as:

- agony over the chances of the baby's survival and the quality of his future;
- guilt and loss of self-esteem at her failure to give birth to a healthy, normal baby; and
- grief for the lost baby whom she will never bring to term (Kaplan & Mason, 1960; Caplan *et al.*, 1965).

The mother of a preterm baby cannot escape the feeling of guilt, even if it is likely to be illogical – it must be 'her fault'. She may believe that to give birth prematurely is a punishment for something she has done or failed to do during pregnancy, or even in her past life; like the mother, for instance, who perceived her newborn baby's fatal cardiac abnormality as merited punishment for a previous termination of pregnancy.

There does not seem to be any way of sparing the mother of a preterm or very sick baby feelings of guilt. Even if the cause is known and explained to her, she will find another source of self-condemnation. It might help her to know that this is a feeling she shares with almost all mothers of babies in NUs. Nevertheless, it must not be forgotten that behind her guilt there may be a very real need. If maternal stress during pregnancy is one of the factors influencing premature labour, and if smoking or inadequate diet are reasons for failure to thrive *in utero*, then the mother is justified in feeling guilty. She will perceive that it is her failure to care for herself in pregnancy that has brought her to this state. Her personal or socio-economic problems need to be identified if she is to be helped.

All women are different in their ability to cope with motherhood. This ability (or lack of it) will depend on their own experiences as children, their age, their emotional maturity, the support they receive from their family, their partner and the community (Carter, 1974). Above all, the mother of the fragile baby needs the support of the neonatal team. A judgmental attitude at this time could be very damaging to her future relationship with her baby; she needs to be accepted as she is, with all her resentment, her anger and her guilt.

Inertia

'It was hard to live day by day with such fear inside me ... A great effort was made to establish a rapport between parents and child.' (Béatrice)

The sight of the apathetic mother sitting by the side of an incubator, peering at her baby through the Perspex, is one of the saddest aspects of the NICU, and one of the most frequently seen. The mother looks drained of energy, helpless and hopeless, and this is indeed exactly how she feels. However, she can use this time of watching and waiting and put it to good effect by getting to know her baby.

The frail appearance of the VLBW baby is intimidating to parents; some are so afraid of him they hesitate to touch him at all. Others will try their utmost to elicit a response from a very immature baby who is quite incapable of interaction at this stage (see Chapter 8). As well as *Born Too Early*, the booklet *This is Your Baby*, explaining the abilities and limitations of preterm infants, can help the mother in her first interactions with her baby (Sparshott, 1989c). She can keep her own observation chart and make a note of his behaviour, and what comforting actions he seems to like (Fig. 9.1). If the baby is very preterm, she can start in a small way by gently touching his hand, and little by little increase this stimulation to stroking, observing his reactions all the time.

One of the difficulties the mother is likely to encounter is a lack of synchrony with regard to eye-to-eye contact. Since this is very important to her, she will try to engage the attention of her preterm infant long before he is ready to maintain this sort of response for any length of time – indeed, sometimes before he can even open his eyes; she is like a child trying to prize open the eyes of a kitten. Activity of this nature is likely to be counterproductive; the more she coaxes, the less likely he is to return her gaze for long.

The state of consciousness of the preterm baby is important, as we have seen; he needs all the periods of deep sleep he can get. The mother can watch her baby sleep, and learn to read his sleep cycle. When he is restless, she can help him to relax by using 'containment'; this is particularly satisfying as it is the nearest she can get to returning her baby to the womb – she encapsulates him in her hands. 'Kangaroo care' as described in Chapter 7 will give her an even closer contact with her baby, but this is only advisable in cases where the infant's condition is stable. Great sensitivity is needed if the mothers of ventilated babies are not to be so terrified by the ventilator and monitors that the good effects of skin-to-skin contact are negated.

Once the sleep/wake cycle of the individual baby is understood by parents, and they have been shown the signals he uses to express his needs, and when they have come to terms with his limitations as an

Observation Chart for Parents

Date: *Example*

My baby's name is: *Mary Devon*

She is *14* days old and her gestational age is: *28 weeks + 2 days*

This is what she likes:

To hear me talk to her
To have her hand held
To lie on her front with her head to the right
To have a rolled blanket to lie against

This is how she behaves:

She looks towards me
She holds my finger
She appears relaxed
She sleeps

This is what she does not like:

A sheepskin
To come out of the incubator
To lie on her side
To be stroked when asleep

This is how she behaves:

She crawls off it
Her toe temperature drops Her heart rate slows
She fidgets
She fidgets and makes faces and sometimes she cries

This is what I like to do for her:

Change her nappy
Clean her mouth

These are things I need help with:

Tube feeding
Turning her over (I get the wires tangled!)

Tomorrow I hope to be here at (time):

11.00 and 18.00 for nursing care

Fig. 9.1 Example of an observation chart for parents. (From Sparshott, 1989c.)

immature being, parents can make daily use of the chart shown in Fig. 9.1 to record for themselves how their baby is progressing, and how far they can engage his attention without him becoming too tired. They can also record for the nurses everything they have observed that appears particularly stressful for their own baby, and what consolation techniques seem to give the most pleasure. The mother may even see for herself that to resist touching her baby when he is resting is a positive and beneficial act. In these ways she gains some control over the situation, and can feel she is necessary for her baby's well-being. As the baby matures and improves in health, so both parents will be able to take pleasure in the passing of milestones, and feel that they themselves were instrumental in his so doing.

Many NUs keep diaries to record the baby's progress; this is particularly valuable if the parents live at some distance and cannot visit frequently. These diaries can contain photographs, and comments made by everyone involved – nursing and medical staff, siblings and the parents themselves. The diaries, as well as the progress charts, can also provide a personal memento for the family later on when the child is safely home, and can even prove to be a comfort if the outcome is not so happy, and the baby does not survive.

Grief

'I felt terribly frustrated by the feeling of emptiness, the failure of my pregnancy, the minuteness of the baby I had been allowed to see only for a moment; in such conditions it is difficult to feel like a mother, and the separation was for me as brutal as it was unexpected.' (Béatrice)

Enormous tasks confront a woman who is already shocked and bewildered, and weary from a premature delivery. She is overwhelmed by double-mourning; as well as the grief she feels for the imagined baby who never materialised, the mother must face the possibility that the real baby might die. She must adapt herself to the idea of her baby's prematurity, and then restore him to life again in her imagination, and frequently she is reluctant to offer love to a being who might soon disappear for ever. Nurses should be alert to the mother of the very sick baby who appears to be rejecting him; it may be that she is simply afraid to become too close.

If the baby is very fragile it is often impossible to predict whether he will live or die. Sophisticated life-support techniques have made it possible to be optimistic, and it is often best to assure parents that babies are more resilient than they look; certainly many small babies do well. There are likely to be setbacks, and parents may have to face many disappointments; but they should be led to understand that babies often take two steps forward to one step back. Also parents are sensitive to the way information is given; one father observed that the positive approach of 'he will only be in the box for six or seven weeks' gave him more confidence in the future than 'he will be in the box at least six or seven weeks'. Nurses should remember to phrase sentences optimistically (Morris, 1994).

Certainly nothing will diminish the tension of a long period of uncertainty, but after a while parents can gain a little confidence and begin to hope, especially when the baby begins to communicate by means of a concentrated gaze at a face, or by turning his head to the sound of a voice.

Acceptance

'Now Chloé really existed for us ... I marvelled at this little girl, so pretty, so fragile, and at the same time so strong ... I kept telling her how much we loved her and longed for her to come home.' (Béatrice)

The imaginary baby of prenatal dreams gradually merges into the real one; once the parents can see the baby as 'their own' they will cease to mourn for the baby that never was and will accept the baby that exists. Parents can be helped to recognise their baby's identity if he is referred to by name, and his gender is remembered – babies are not neuter and should never be referred to as 'it'. Identity can also be established by reference to special characteristics, such as long fingers, nicely shaped ears, preference for a certain posture. If at first they are unable to hold and caress him, the provision of cuddly toys in the incubator (but not too many and not too large!), cassettes of nursery rhymes, music boxes and little books will help to make a preterm infant a 'person' for his parents, and when he is stronger they can dress him in his own clothes.

Free access to visitors at the parents' discretion will help to render the atmosphere more natural. The embarrassment some parents feel at having to explain to friends that they have a baby who is 'not normal' will be dissipated if these same friends are allowed to see the baby in his incubator. Parents can air their knowledge by explaining the ventilatory and monitoring systems, and have even been heard to boast that their baby is 'the smallest!' Pride in their baby can sometimes be encouraged by suggesting to parents that they are, indeed, privileged to see him at this time. How many mothers can watch their baby develop and grow from 24 weeks of the pregnancy?

All the mother's feelings of revulsion, fear and guilt will be compounded by a sense of inadequacy at her baby's dependence for survival, not on her own competence, but on strangers – the neonatal staff. Understanding the importance of her role as the comforter and consoler of her baby will help the mother to feel less inadequate. Her confidence will be restored as she begins to participate and then take over his nursing care.

This process must be conducted at the mother's own speed. If she is nervous at first, she should not be forced or expected to handle her baby (Redman, 1993); her reluctance to do so will only increase her sense of guilt. The nurse can begin to show her simple nursing care procedures, such as cleaning the mouth, and as she grows in confidence she can do more. If she goes home before her baby, procedures such as the daily toilet or bath can be left for her to do when she comes to visit, and she can make a note of these on the chart (Fig. 9.1). Some NUs have a notice board on the wall beside each cot or incubator where parents can write down their visiting times, and what care they wish to give the baby. By the time she takes her baby home, the mother should have established a routine with the nursing staff whereby she is the one who dictates when things are done; this will restore her sense that the baby belongs to her.

The father

'I soon realised that fathers are not supposed to have emotions.' (Hay, 1990)

The role of the father within the family remains stereotyped to a certain extent; in spite of changes within recent years, shared parenting is still a rare phenomenon. Sociological studies of parenthood suggest that though fathers are prepared to 'help', the main responsibility for the child is still taken by the mother; it seems that fathers are making their contribution to their children's development through 'play' (Beail, 1983).

There are a number of problems that are specific to the father:

- Whatever he feels, he is expected to maintain his masculine role.
- He is faced with disruption of the home.
- He is responsible for maintaining the household routine – other children to keep happy, grandparents to reassure, friends to keep informed, etc.
- He may be ashamed at feelings of inadequacy and actual fear of the baby.
- He may feel anger at his inability to control the situation.
- He must contend with the practical responsibilities associated with the birth of a baby (such as registration) which may be complicated by a premature birth.
- He may have financial worries.
- Sometimes, he may be jealous of losing the attention of his wife or partner.

For the father, as well as for the mother, the routine of life has been disrupted by the birth of the preterm baby; he sees his partner absorbed by her own guilt and anxiety, while for him 'life must go on'. He must work, cook meals, take the dog for walks and look after the other children while his partner is in hospital; the presence of a large and boisterous dog can itself be a bone of contention between partners to whose lifestyle has been added a fragile being requiring the utmost protection.

Most mothers need the support of their partners, but this is a strain on the father. Advertisements in magazines and on television still tend to emphasise a macho image (although fortunately this is beginning to change). The father may feel the need to express his own feelings of sorrow and fear, but be prevented from doing so by seeing his role as one who must be stalwart. 'Not once did anyone ask me how I was feeling,' said Hay (1990), 'and I would have loved for someone to have said just once "and how are you?" ' The father can easily be forgotten as a person who also needs support within the 'holding' environment of the NU, though his role as manager of crises and master of the situation may be taken for granted. Concern is concentrated mainly on mother and baby; but very often it is the father who has the first contact with his baby, as the mother may still be recovering from the effects of the delivery, or caesarian section.

By this early visiting, and the questions he has to ask in his role as go-between for the baby and mother, the father may feel a proprietary interest from the first. On the other hand, he can see his usefulness reduced to that of a messenger, fit only to run errands between mother and child (Voyer, 1986). He may also feel his loyalties are divided on who needs him most, the fragile infant alone with strangers or the mother whom he must try to reassure (Voyer, 1986; Shellabarger & Thompson, 1993). Although the father is not tormented by guilt at failing to fulfil the function of successfully bringing forth a child, he may well experience guilt at his failure to protect mother and baby when both appear to be in physical danger, and this may turn to helpless anger. It needs great understanding for the father to share the mother's feelings of guilt, and failure to do this may make him insensitive to her need for reassurance.

The father is generally not so intimidated by technical equipment as the mother, and may find his interest in the life support systems a means of relating to his baby. Although description of these should not be forced on parents whose main concern is the well-being of their child, the caregiver may find it helpful to attract the initial interest of the father by showing how each piece of equipment is helping to maintain the life of the baby (Vine, 1995). (Of course stereotyping is not exclusive to the fathers; most mothers are quite capable of understanding monitoring equipment. On the whole, however, the future well-being of the baby is their first priority.)

The father can be intimidated by the baby himself, a fact that may not be easy for him to accept. Inhibited by his masculine role, the father doubts whether he can provide adequate care, so he holds back (Hawthorne *et al.*, 1978). Fathers frequently complain that their hands are too big, and they are afraid of hurting the child. This is a pity, because many men are skilled at and sensitive in handling their babies, and become as adept as the mothers. Many fathers get immense pleasure out of feeding and nappy changing, and hold back only because they assume this to be 'women's work'. The early involvement of fathers in nursing care should be warmly encouraged, however, as there is some evidence that fathers who interact with their newborn preterm infants will tend to continue in a good relationship; follow-up studies have shown that this early attachment endures (Richards, 1983).

If the father feels a high sense of involvement, it eases the burden for the mother and the whole family relationship will be influenced (Jacques *et al.*, 1983); the sharing of tasks and experiences is also likely to be beneficial when the baby is eventually discharged, since he, too, will become accustomed to attentions from both parents.

Siblings

It is the policy in most NUs nowadays to encourage visiting by brothers and sisters, and to establish the whole family as a unit from the beginning. Sometimes it is not easy for neonatal staff; little children get under foot, make a noise, get fractious and, worst of all, are full of curiosity and like to touch and pull at wires and tubes. On the other hand visiting the baby with their parents is beneficial to siblings, and family visiting of this kind usually works very well. The other children are able to adjust themselves to the idea of a little brother or sister, without having to support the prolonged disappearances of Mother. A booklet *Special Care Babies*, explaining the NU to children, can help them feel welcome and involved ('Althea', 1986). The sitting room provided for the parents should also facilitate the accommodation of siblings when they become bored with the nurseries, and many NUs provide boxes of books and toys, or a Wendy House, to keep them amused. They can be helped to feel that they are participating by being encouraged to bring toys for the baby, or drawings they have done specially for him. Since most little children like to draw, a supply of coloured pencils and scrap paper can keep them happy, and if afterwards their artistic efforts are placed in the cot or incubator, or even displayed on a board reserved for this purpose, the siblings will be helped to feel a necessary part of life on the unit.

It is always advisable for the nursing staff to remember that there may be brothers and sisters at home; a mother whose visits are irregular may not be rejecting her new baby, but harassed by problems of baby-sitting. If for some reason the mother does not wish to bring her other children into hospital with her, or at least not for all her visits, the social worker may be able to help her to resolve this problem.

'The child "belongs" to his parents, not to neonatal staff; one must have the strength to claim one's place and one's rights, and refuse to be treated as incapable just because one isn't a doctor.' (Béatrice)

There was no happy ending to the story of Béatrice and Chloé; after months of alternate happiness and great suffering for her parents, Chloé died. Towards the end of her life she was moved from one hospital, where she had prospered, to another one that was more 'institutional' and less aware of her emotional needs. The circumstances of her death led her mother to say: 'Premature babies are also individuals gifted with sense and sensitivity; I am now convinced that their lives are intimately linked with the environment that is created for them. Chloé died because one day she ceased to struggle against an environment which could not give her the desire and the will to live...'

Chapter 10
Caring for the Caregivers

The pain of inflicting pain

The prospect of suffering which the observer is unable to relieve can have a contradictory effect; it is hard to look on and be unable to help. Frustrated in the instinctive desire to reach out to the victim, the observer may either feel bitter resentment, or turn aside. But caregivers in the NICU are unable to turn aside. Even if in the circumstances doctors and nurses can rationalise the action, it is unnatural to inflict pain on a newborn baby. In some ways it can be seen as inflicting a form of punishment on the child – the price he must pay for survival. The caregivers are determined to save the child, by force, in a battle where the contestants are very unevenly matched.

When all hope of saving him is gone, doctors and nurses try to supress murderous feelings when they watch the prolonged agony of the dying baby. They silently beg him to die, and are bitterly ashamed of their relief when at last, by doing so, he releases them from the pressures of guilt and inadequacy. The hollow-eyed stare, the feeble whimper or 'silent cry' of the severely ill newborn infant are harder to bear than the indignant yelling of the well baby:

> 'We have developed many tactics for dealing with feelings of guilt and inadequacy. Irritation, denial and withdrawal are the most common. Everyone close to a patient in prolonged pain battles with conflicting tendencies to approach and withdraw.' (Melzack & Wall, 1988)

There is no way that caregivers in the NICU can avoid stress; the day-to-day events in such a place make that inevitable. Nurses experience feelings of rivalry, anger and hostility towards parents, whose care they see as inadequate – they would do so much better themselves! Parents may find students more sympathetic than experienced nurses, because the work is new to them and they, too, may find things intimidating. Very often there is a tendency for all staff (except the allocated or named nurse) to avoid the parents of a dying baby (Bender & Swan-Parente,

1983); this is partly because they remember hopes that have been given in the past, now not likely to be realised.

> 'The physicians, surgeons and associated health professionals who take part in the treatment of pain are first of all human beings and therefore subject to the same pressures of guilt and inadequacy as other people.' (Melzack & Wall, 1988)

The stresses discussed in this chapter are the stresses peculiar to the NICU, where so much is demanded of so few. Stress is necessary to keep the adrenaline flowing; without stress we would become lethargic and bored. Most of us think we would love a peaceful life, but though periods of quiet on the NICU delight us and give us a chance to give the babics the holistic care we feel they deserve, all will recognise, I am sure, the feeling of lassitude that accompanies a prolonged period of calm – and the quality of work is not always improved.

The line between what we will support day-by-day and what suddenly becomes unendurable is a fine one; but once that line is passed, we are likely to find ourselves on the downward spiral towards 'burn out', and all the complications this state creates for us and the people around us.

> 'To offer the kind of care that is required in a maternity hospital makes a great demand on staff and raises problems that go far beyond issues of technical expertise. Deep feelings and conflicts may be aroused for the staff and opportunities need to be created where these can be expressed and examined.' (Richards, 1978)

The Neonatal Intensive Care Unit

A multiplicity of factors leads to the high rate of stress-related illness, low morale and absenteeism termed 'burn out' in the NICU. Amongst these factors are: 'Rage, frustration, envy and other very strong feelings as well as the moral and ethical dilemmas of working on such a unit' (Bender & Swan-Parente, 1983). 'Unit politics' can be responsible for many ills; NICUs where there is rivalry or conflict between disciplines and grades will not function well. No matter how competent the individual, there will be a lack of integrity at the centre. Most important of all, the relationship existing between neonatal staff will have an effect on parents and babies:

> 'Until they come to terms with their own feelings about the job it may be difficult for nurses and doctors in neonatal units to understand parental attitudes and to cope with parents' feelings.' (Jaques *et al.*, 1983)

As well as problems of their own associated with their disciplines, professional carers have problems with each other. Ancient resentments arising from archaic hierarchical structures still survive (Fig. 10.1), and can be seen occasionally in the 'kick the dog' syndrome. This is a chain of events starting with the consultant criticising the sister for the way her ward is run; red in the face, but not daring to reply, she scolds the staff nurse for failing to maintain order; the staff nurse then upbraids the SHO for being a clumsy ass; the SHO informs the student midwife that she is completely incapable; and the student midwife (with no dog to kick)

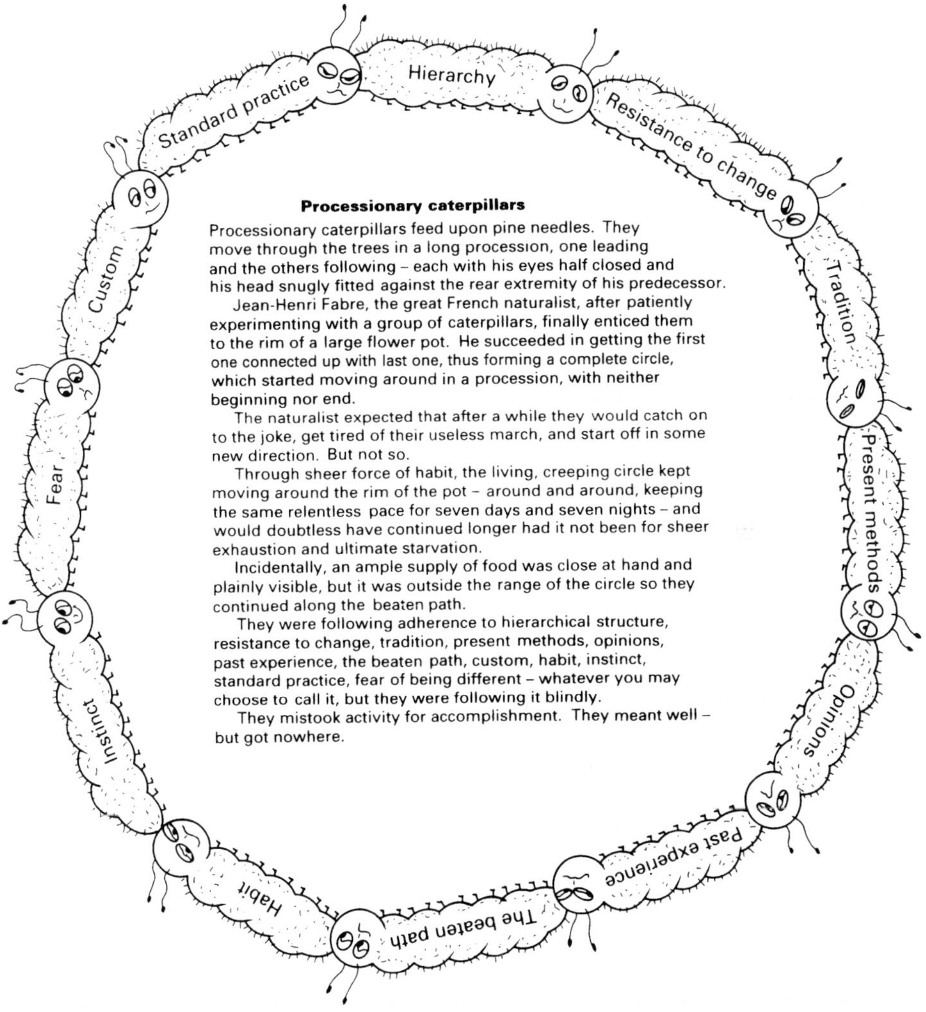
Hierarchy
Resistance to change
Tradition
Present methods
Opinions
Past experience
The beaten path
Habit
Instinct
Fear
Custom
Standard practice
Processionary caterpillars
Processionary caterpillars feed upon pine needles. They move through the trees in a long procession, one leading and the others following – each with his eyes half closed and his head snugly fitted against the rear extremity of his predecessor.
Jean-Henri Fabre, the great French naturalist, after patiently experimenting with a group of caterpillars, finally enticed them to the rim of a large flower pot. He succeeded in getting the first one connected up with last one, thus forming a complete circle, which started moving around in a procession, with neither beginning nor end.
The naturalist expected that after a while they would catch on to the joke, get tired of their useless march, and start off in some new direction. But not so.
Through sheer force of habit, the living, creeping circle kept moving around the rim of the pot – around and around, keeping the same relentless pace for seven days and seven nights – and would doubtless have continued longer had it not been for sheer exhaustion and ultimate starvation.
Incidentally, an ample supply of food was close at hand and plainly visible, but it was outside the range of the circle so they continued along the beaten path.
They were following adherence to hierarchical structure, resistance to change, tradition, present methods, opinions, past experience, the beaten path, custom, habit, instinct, standard practice, fear of being different – whatever you may choose to call it, but they were following it blindly.
They mistook activity for accomplishment. They meant well – but got nowhere.

Fig. 10.1 Processionary caterpillars. (Courtesy of Columbia/HCA Healthcare Corporation, adapted from the *Humana Care Manual*, 1982.)

goes into the linen cupboard to cry. This strict hierarchical system of ward management which allowed the dog to be kicked still exists in some NUs, but has tended to give way to more relaxed systems which emphasise closer collaboration between the disciplines.

Some outlet for the relief of feelings is necessary. Kicking dogs will only help in the short term; individual conferences or group discussions can be of more permanent value. Bender and Swan-Parente (1983) recommended that there should be a 'forum for expression – a neutral territory in which everyone can contribute equally irrespective of hierarchical structures'. One unit with a problem of hierarchical antagonism started a Neonatal Journal/Discussion Club, which entailed members of the team meeting for an hour once a month to discuss a paper, presented by a speaker, that could be circulated in advance. In this particular unit the Journal Club proved a very successful way of bringing people together and integrating them as a team of carers (Fletcher, 1979).

Similar schemes have been developed in other units, with the same success; others, however, have found that after initial enthusiasm, group meetings are poorly attended. But even if interdisciplinary meetings are difficult to organise, regular peer group meetings to discuss specific unit problems and ways in which to cope with them can be a valuable method of relieving stress (Hannon, 1993).

Nurses and managers

'I could lie down like a tired child/And weep away the life of care,' said Shelley – and how we would agree with him! Many NICUs, even prestigious ones, have problems in recruiting nurses, and many nurses leave after only a short time of service. The physical and emotional pressure experienced, the apparent lack of respect and recognition, a salary incompatible with responsibility, and chronic staff shortages are the main factors contributing to this.

Yet if some leave after a short time, many neonatal nurses love the work they do and remain in this field all their working lives, accepting the rough with the smooth:

> 'The intensity and complexity of the intensive care necessary to help preterm infants survive draws staff with uncompromising dedication to this work.' (Als, 1986)

Uncompromising dedication is often abused, however, and administrators should remember that:

> '... stress will be exacerbated by a high work load and insufficient staff, and senior staff should watch that high motivation, however

commendable, does not lead staff to work grossly in excess of their normal duty.' (Third Maternity Services Advisory Committee Report, 1985)

Moreover, idealism, commitment, enthusiasm, energy and patience, the very qualities that constitute 'uncompromising dedication', are those most likely to lead to burn out.

A list of the causes of stress among neonatal nurses shows that shortage of staff is one of the principal nightmares (Table 10.1). Nursing staffing levels in many units fall short of recommended standards, and this has serious implications. Some regional and trust administrators seem to take these implications on board, but many others are less positive, some even denying the existence of a problem (Redshaw & Harris, 1995). Lack of qualified staff means either that nurses are undertaking a heavy workload, or that nurses without the appropriate training are being asked to take responsibility for very ill babies 'because there is no one else'. Response to a questionnaire sent to neonatal units in 1989 showed that lack of support from administration was a common cause of stress; nurses felt that their work was not understood by management: 'they think all we do is feed babies!' was one comment (Sparshott, 1989b). This lack of understanding seems to be shown in a grading system which has no respect for special skills, and where promotion, until very recently, has only been possible by moving out of the clinical field, leading to a competitive environment that may be detrimental to good team work (Patton Dunbar, 1995). Fortunately, good managers are awake to this problem: 'I feel very strongly about my ability to help where necessary and not spend 100% of my time on paper work. This in turn helps to relieve stress, also creating the right atmosphere in the team, nurses and all doctors included' (manager's response to 1989 questionnaire).

One thing seems certain; a clear and direct leadership, and the presentation of a clear and direct policy, are essential to the well-being of a neonatal unit. Neonatal staff must be able to trust their leader, and they must have a common purpose and philosophy. If the unit policy is vague and staff are given no sense of direction, it will lead to feelings of insecurity and mistrust. A sense of well-being is instilled from above, and the opposite is also true; the Greeks (as always) have a saying for this: 'the rotten fish stinks from the head'.

Nurses and nurses

The ambiance of the nurses' own unit plays a large part in their well-being. The NUs which appear from the 1989 questionnaire to have the most positive approach to their work are those where a good relation-

Table 10.1   Stress factors of nurses in the NICU.

Causes of stress	Relief of stress
NICU staff	
Lack of trained nursing and medical staff	Adequately trained neonatal staff
Lack of support from administration	Clear nursing policies
Fear of litigation	Having a nursing officer responsible for unit
Responsibility for lives of fragile babies ⎱	Unit counsellor, psychotherapist, mutual
Terminal care ⎰	support, support group
The moral and ethical dilemmas experienced	Consultant showing concern for nursing staff
	Inter-disciplinary unit meetings
Need for technical expertise	Mentor system for new staff
Need to make quick decisions at times of crisis ⎱	Approachability of Unit Sister
Inflexibility (petty procedures) ⎰	
Inexperienced staff responsible for fragile babies ⎱	Rotation through unit
Working only in intensive care ⎰	
Being asked to work in other areas	Patient allocation as opposed to job allocation
Disruptive shifts and rotations ⎱	Overtime payments made promptly
	Time off in lieu granted at time agreed by nurse
⎰	Ability to choose holiday
Low status and pay	Opportunity to pursue research or projects
Lack of opportunities for further education due to lack of funds	Study days, conferences, in-service training, sabbatical leave
Friction between nurses and inexperienced SHOs	Presence of a nurse practitioner
Working with locum doctor	Support from senior medical staff
Preoccupation with non-nursing tasks	Presence of ward clerk
General stress of intensive care nursing ⎱	Participating in social events
⎰	Seeing babies after discharge
NICU	
Lack of privacy ⎱	Opportunity to get away from unit during working hours
	Adequate accommodation for parents
Heat and noise of the unit ⎱	Rest room for nurses
	Provision of beverages on the unit
⎰	Provision for cooking light meals
Unsuitable uniforms	Wearing sandals and light dresses
Equipment breakdown	Unit technician to service monitors
Lack of storage space	A well-designed unit
Inadequate laundry facilities	Well-organised domestic services

(Adapted and extended from Bender & Swann-Parente, 1983; Chiswick & Roberton, 1987; Sparshott, 1989b. Reproduced by kind permission of *Nursing Times* where first published 18 October 1989.)

ship exists within the team; sporting events, organisation of evenings out together and enjoyment of mutual interests are popular. Nurses agree, too, that it is best not to let the sun go down on anger: 'any grudges with each other and we go into the linen cupboard and sort it out without prying ears!' – oh! what dramas those linen cupboards have seen!

One of the ways of relieving stress most frequently mentioned in responses to the 1989 questionnaire was the opportunity for further education, for participation at conferences, and for carrying out research; even if lengthy periods of study leave are not possible, half-day or day release for seminars has been found to help nurses retain their confidence (Walker, 1982). It is clear that nurses who work in the field of neonatology want to improve their skills, and should be encouraged to do so. Nor is it uneconomical to set aside funds for this, as opportunities for training and subsequently promotion will also ensure that qualified nurses remain in the specialty (Third Maternity Services Advisory Committee Report, 1985).

Belonging to relevant professional organisations is also helpful, since as well as providing opportunities for further education in organising local conferences and study days, they put nurses and midwives in touch with each other. It is stimulating to share experiences with colleagues from other hospitals – and it is salutary to learn that others have problems too!

There are stress and counselling services available in some Regional Health Authorities – effective counselling is dependent on personality, however, and neonatal nurses should find the person who they feel is the most appropriate to their needs; this may be a psychotherapist, hospital chaplain, or even their own unit manager. The Royal College of Nursing also supplies a Counselling and Advisory Service (Appendix 4). Nurses appear most comfortable when they depend on each other for support, however:

> 'By sharing our experiences we considerably lessen the stress, manage to keep things in perspective, and in so doing improve our efficiency and ability to care for the babies.' (response to 1989 questionnaire)

It is true that the burden of supporting parents in their grief for their dying baby, as well as coping with one's own sadness, is greatly lightened by the sympathy and understanding of colleagues.

At the Neonatal Nurses Association annual conference held in Liverpool in 1995, Melodie Chenevert, 'Pro-Nurse' from Gaithersburg, USA, spoke of the 'nurses of Oz' who, not having a yellow brick road to follow, needed to find a sense of direction of their own. She believes nurses suffer from an unmerited lack of self-esteem. She reminded us that, in Oz, the scarecrow was searching for a brain, the lion was searching for courage, and the tin man was searching for a heart; but all they needed to do to supply themselves with these qualities was to pin them on themselves like medals – in other words, they had them all the time, without realising it!

Nurses and parents

One undesirable side-effect of the dedication of neonatal nurses to their work can be an unwitting rivalry between staff and parents. The over-possessive nurse may dominate the mother to such an extent that a false mother/daughter relationship is created between them; this can only be damaging to the baby. The mother who remains a child herself will find difficulty in appropriating the responsibility for her own child (Als, 1986). Conversely, competition may lead to a spirit of aggression in the mother, and this may make ominous waves throughout the unit; other parents become involved, and soon there is a miasma of resentment and ill-feeling. Even more dangerous is the possessive nurse who so organises her work load that it is *she* who baths the baby, gives him his feed and all his care, ignoring the only available visiting times for the parents.

'Providing effective care without usurping the parental role is perhaps the most difficult task that faces a neonatal unit.' (Richards, 1983)

When young parents appear to be feckless, nurses may fear for the future of the baby, and show their disapproval by sharp criticism and reproach. This is likely to be counterproductive, as the 'fecklessness' may be due to (and is always associated with) a dislike and fear of 'Authority' which would, by the nurse's attitude, appear to be justified. Of course the nurse is responsible, with others, for seeing that the baby is not sent home into danger; but sometimes the stress of witnessing the long struggle to live of a very fragile infant has a maturing effect on the young mother, and the support and approval of the neonatal team will go a long way towards reinforcing this maturity.

Doctors

House Officers in training for general practice frequently dread their term in neonatal intensive care, since this is likely to involve them in working long hours without rest. A report issued in 1989 by the British Postgraduate Medical Federation found that junior staff in paediatrics work the longest hours, are the busiest at night, and are the most likely to have sleep interrupted, than staff in any other speciality (Dowie, 1989). In other fields involving air and road traffic, where accidents have occurred due to tired personnel, legislation has led to restriction of working hours. In spite of recent improvements in policy, doctors continue to work long hours, and reforms are slow. Many doctors feel they have little opportunity to complain or state their case. They fear that complaints may damage their reputation within the profession and their chances of advancement, and indeed these fears have not always proved unfounded. Senior physicians can still be heard to recall the old days when they, too, were required to work long hours: 'and if I could do it, so can they'. But these physicians forget that modern technology has increased the responsibilities of doctors, as it has decreased the risk of mortality, and reduced the gestational age at which life can be saved.

Junior doctors' hours have been reduced, but this has led to the problem of a work load that has not diminished, but remains the same. This problem would be relieved if there was an increase in the number of neonatologists, and if some of the tasks undertaken up to now by junior doctors were performed by other professionals (McKee *et al.*, 1991).

Evidence of burn-out has also been recorded in senior medical staff, and can be seen in over reliance on junior staff, inflexibility, resistance to change, and sometimes even a reluctance to visit the unit. Consultant paediatricians and neonatalogists have heavy responsibilities which cannot be shared; they are the ones who ultimately confirm life and death decisions, and must discuss with parents the consequences of long-term handicap. As with obstetricians, the success or failure of consultant paediatricians is constantly open to public scrutiny (Walker, 1982). The rotation of junior staff means that the consultant neonatologist is constantly faced with the responsibility of training a new team, and an inevitable drop in quality of care when inexperienced staff are in the process of learning; neonatal registrars take much of this responsibility, but ultimately they, too, must move on and be replaced. Delegation is, however, a possibility for the consultant; but is not always easy for the neonatal nurse.

Nurse practitioners

There is conflict between the need of NICUs for experienced and dedicated staff, and the idea that the primary function of junior doctors is to complete their training. Since the sharp division of roles between nurse and doctor often causes friction when an experienced neonatal nurse works alongside an inexperienced SHO, a more flexible integration of staff would be of benefit to babies (Chiswick & Roberton, 1987). Some neonatal nurses could, with their bedside experience, be trained to take over such procedures as intubation, sampling and measuring arterial blood gasses, adjusting ventilator settings, inserting peripheral lines and arterial catheters, draining pneumothoraces and treating hypovolaemic shock. These skills could be used in district and regional hospitals, relieving the pressure on doctors, and the necessity for the transfer of babies elsewhere. Chiswick and Roberton made the following propositions:

- **Introduction of ward policy** – to serve as a guide for the management of babies with various disorders. This guide, decided jointly by medical and nursing staff, should combine elements of traditional nursing care with medical treatment.
- **Continuity of care** – individual nurses on each shift care for particular babies. Experienced neonatal nurses should work outside the traditional system together with medical staff, providing continuity of care between shifts.
- **Participation in ward rounds** – under these circumstances joint ward rounds would permit more critical planning of a baby's total needs and are intellectually stimulating and educational for all staff.
- **Joint medical and nursing representation** – intensive care units require the services of neonatal nurse teachers, and these posts should be considered senior prestigious positions. (Chiswick & Roberton, 1987)

Most of these propositions have been implemented by the introduction of the roles of named nurse, nurse practitioner and clinical nurse teacher – and in some cases they have been implemented only to be withdrawn again in the present climate of 'save money, no matter what the cost in quality'. It has been argued that the hierarchical structure of the NU might be damaged by the introduction of yet another level of competence into the system, in the shape of the neonatal nurse practitioner. On the whole, however, this role has been well received; it is seen as a career prospect in a specialism that otherwise offers limited opportunities for advancement, and it is perceived by other nurses as offering a quality of care that is more skilled, because it is more consistent, than that offered by a junior doctor (Hall *et al.*, 1992). The role of neonatal nurse practitioner is still young, and there have been some teething problems – if female, she appears to be seen by many consultants as 'there to take the pressure off the SHOs'; in other words, just another handmaiden!

Nurses, doctors and pain relief

Because of rotation systems and the exigencies of training, delicate procedures are often undertaken by doctors in the process of learning, who leave the unit as soon as they have become proficient, in order to make way for others to learn. The procedures listed in Chapter 6 are many of them difficult to do and require considerable dexterity. Three months is not very long for the gaining of proficiency in such skills; SHOs are aware of this and are naturally anxious to succeed. This means that they are often reluctant to seek help from the registrar, but will try over and over again in the hope that practice will make perfect. Many units make a rule that after the third failed attempt, SHOs must send for help, but understandably they do not wish to admit defeat, particularly at night when it means disturbing the duty registrar.

The problem of the handling of babies by SHOs in the process of gaining experience in a field of medicine they do not intend to follow has caused friction on many units. It also causes distress to the doctors themselves: 'All I ever seem to do is hurt babies', one caring SHO was heard to say. A specialist phlebotomist can be of great help in the taking of routine blood samples, but obviously cannot always be available. Many neonatal nurses feel that such routine procedures as venepuncture could be performed by an experienced nurse. At the present time, nurses undertake the siting of i.v. cannulae in only a few units in the UK; in Europe and the USA they commonly do this work. If practice makes perfect, then not only the neonatal nurse practitioner but also the experienced neonatal nurse seem the people most likely to perform venepuncture successfully; time would be saved if the baby did not have to wait for the return of the doctor called away for an emergency; nights 'on call' would be more tolerable if the doctor were not continually disturbed for routine procedures. There would be less damage and wastage of fragile veins, and therefore less suffering for the baby (Sparshott, 1989b). The most important way of reducing the pain of traumatic procedures for the baby, then, is to ensure that such procedures should be skilfully done.

The nurse, helping the doctor in the performance of such procedures as lumbar puncture and intubation, must play the part of the baby's advocate. The way a nurse conveys that a baby is in pain may influence the doctor's subsequent actions. A flat announcement 'I know he is in pain!' does not justify the administration of analgesia from the doctor's point of view. He or she may feel obliged to order the prescription more to keep the nurse quiet than to relieve the baby. The nurse also starts on the wrong footing by assuming the role of 'the one who knows' (how? feminine instinct? masculine gut-feeling?) and if this 'knowledge' is rejected, the rejection will be seen as a personal affront (Als, 1986). This is a game in which the baby plays a poor third party.

When it is a question of abstaining from the performance of a traumatic procedure, or the administration of analgesia, it will be more helpful if the nurse can give cogent clinical reasons for so doing. A precise demonstration of the physiological and behavioural responses that have given rise to the claim of knowledge is far more likely to persuade the doctor that a medical decision is being made on a clinical basis, not an emotional one. The pain management chart (Table 6.2) and the pain scoring system NIPS (Table 5.1) or DSVNI (Appendix 2: Sparshott, 1996) can be useful in this context.

'It should not be forgotten that our medical colleagues are human beings also, that even though they may not show it, sometimes they may feel anything from frustration to despair at lack of success in treating pain ... The way forward is not by demanding that our medical colleagues change prescriptions (or their ways), but by mutual co-operation in facing the challenge of relieving patient suffering.' (Sofaer, 1985)

Education

Education concerning neonatal pain control is neglected. There will be less controversy between medical and nursing staff and consequently less tension if a proper protocol is established for pain management. Doctors, as well as nurses, should be aware of newborn pain responses and have clear guidelines on what actions to take. Doctors employed on units that specialise in the treatment of children in pain should first receive training in such techniques as the installation of a central venous line so that, without traumatising the child, medication can be given over a long period of time (de Bel, 1989). Speaking on paediatric pain in general, McGrath and Unruh propose the following:

- integration of paediatric pain issues into the training of nurses and doctors;
- publication of paediatric studies and reviews in the professional and scientific literature;
- public education about paediatric pain;
- development of educational material for professionals;
- interdisciplinary research. (McGrath & Unruh, 1987)

Ethics and research

On the subject of ethics, there are several questions caregivers should ask themselves, to which the answers are by no means unequivocal:

Question 1

Are caregivers justified in employing pain-relieving drugs, since the effects of the different types of analgesia are still unknown to a certain extent, and since research must involve using them to assess their value? Or conversely, do caregivers have the right to *withold* analgesia in the treatment of pain?

The extent of pain experienced by an infant requiring CMV/IMV, PTV, ECMO, or high-frequency oscillation ventilation has not as yet been established, although all are theoretically traumatic. Ventilated infants may not always require pain relief, but generally the protocol is to prevent pain/distress by the administration of narcotic analgesia. The use of carefully calculated doses of opioid analgesia has now proved its value, and become common practice. Some of the hesitation by doctors to prescribe analgesia in the presence of pain arose from a confusion between drug addiction, dependence and tolerance, but it is now understood that there is no question of subsequent addiction following the treatment of infants, and those who become dependent can be weaned from the drug (Anand *et al.*, 1993) (see Chapter 6). Anxious parents should be reassured that their baby is being made more comfortable, that his pain is being relieved, and that the use of narcotics will not increase the risk of future drug problems (Franck, 1989).

Question 2

Who gives consent for experimental treatment?

Treatment cannot be given against the patient's will, but how can one know the will of a newborn baby, 'an unprotected individual who cannot express a view on the desirability to live' (Bissenden, 1986)? In this case, it is the parents who must give informed consent for any experimental treatment to be given or research to be carried out. Consent must be given 'without duress', which means that no pressure must be brought to bear in order to evoke consent; and 'without fraud', which means that physicians must be truthful about the possible risks and benefits of treatment. In some cases such decisions have to be made quickly, but it is preferable if the parents can have time to discuss the subject between themselves. Decisions taken too quickly may be regretted later, and the parents may resent the medical staff if they feel that pressure has been brought to bear. If this happens, parents may view informed consent as 'a perfunctory activity to fulfil legal requirements', and feel that whatever their wishes, the decision will be taken out of their hands (Schlomann, 1992).

Question 3

Do caregivers have a right to inflict pain in the first place, even for the infant's own eventual well-being?

Non-therapeutic pain research in the NICU does not present ethical problems, since necessary procedures such as vaccination, venepuncture or heel-prick blood sampling have made it possible for researchers to study emotional and physiological reactions to painful stimuli without inflicting further trauma.

If we can only guarantee life, or life of good quality, by the use of traumatic and invasive procedures, then ventilatory support, parenteral nutrition, and all the invasive procedures these entail, are going to be necessary – and by the struggle they make for survival, most babies would seem to be choosing to live, in spite of initial suffering. In 1986, regional centres providing intensive care could offer 50% survival for babies weighing between 750 and 1000 g, and 90% survival between 1000 and 1500 g (Bissenden, 1986). This is probably a modest assessment now.

But what constitutes 'life of good quality'? If 'life is not valuable because of its qualities; it is valuable in itself' (Kuhse & Singer, 1985), does this mean that we should attach infants whose medical conditions are not treatable, such as anencephaly, to life support machinery? When there is a probability of severe handicap due to massive brain damage, must we keep the baby 'artificially' alive by all the technical means available? Some believe not:

> 'To suggest that a person who can achieve a physical and mental age of no more than two, will remain totally dependent, and will be unable to communicate, can have a good quality of life is wrong. It would be an evil person who would support a life of such wretched existence.' (Bissenden, 1986)

There is a difference, however, between allowing an infant to die through denial of life support machinery, and allowing him to die from starvation and neglect:

> 'It is plausible to suppose that newborn infants can feel pain, and prefer not to be in pain; that they can feel cold, and desire not to be cold; that they can feel hungry, and desire not to be hungry. It is, therefore, plausible to suppose that newborn infants have rights to have their pain relieved, and to be kept warm and fed.' (Kuhse & Singer, 1985)

If life support is withdrawn, palliative care must be arranged, not only for the support of the baby, but also for the parents (Brykczynska, 1994).

Question 4

Who makes the final decision – life or death?

Often this task falls to senior medical staff, but for doctors to make such a decision seems contrary to the whole principle of medicine, which is to save life. There are also inherent dangers for professional caregivers who alone decide between life and death; they may see themselves as all-powerful, with their sophisticated techniques. When, having lost the battle, senior doctors feel themselves forced to admit failure, they may try to recapture a sense of power by becoming 'the one who decides, alone and undisputed, between life and death' (Soulé, 1986). Senior medical staff have to try to forget their own position and consider only the interests of the individual baby and his parents. If it is the consultant paediatrician who makes the final decision, he or she is morally obliged to remain to see the outcome, and must not walk away leaving nurses and SHOs to support the parents through their vigil.

If we believe that it is not the doctor but the parents who should make such a decision, is this the time when such a responsibility should be laid upon them? They are confronted by an offspring who is palpably suffering, and whose very existence is a mystery to them. How can they come to any decision, when the future can only be conjectured? There are many parents who beg the doctor to save life, and then regret a decision so hastily made, at a time when they were in no condition to consider all the consequences. Or they hope for a recovery against all odds – and frequently such hopes may be justified, since babies are resilient. In such cases 'seemingly rational parents may not be acting in their own best interest, let alone that of the baby' (Bissenden, 1986).

When neonatal staff and parents are confronted with the choice of continuing a life without future, or withdrawing life support and allowing the baby to die in peace, such decisions should be made with the participation of all concerned. It is important that *everyone* should agree on the course to be taken, and with patience this can usually be achieved:

> 'If the values of the neonatal nurse (reverence for life, dignity, self-determination) are congruent with those of the parents and physician, there can be a harmoniously shared waiting period in which all participants support the decision and one another. In those cases in which the nurse does not share the values and cannot in conscience accept the assignment, conflict may ensue.' (Copp, 1985)

Conflict should not be allowed to ensue; controversy among neonatal staff at such a time can be damaging to the parents, who must live with their memories.

The rights of the foetus

The question of pain experience associated with foetal therapy and surgery is relevant, since we have seen that the foetus is neurologically capable of pain perception from early in the second trimester (Anand & Hickey, 1987) (see Chapter 3). Foetuses of 23 weeks' g.a. and above have shown a hormonal stress response to invasive stimuli *in utero* similar to that which would be mounted by neonates, children and adults (Giannakoulopoulos *et al.*, 1994). Crying has been heard from within the womb, almost always associated with obstetric procedures, and aborted foetuses have been heard to cry from 21 weeks' g.a. (Chamberlain, 1989).

Operating on unanaesthetised foetuses results in autonomic nervous system stimulation, increased hormonal activity and increased motor activity. Invasive surgical techniques in the womb are frequently performed without analgesia; if general anaesthesia is used, it is to provide both maternal and foetal anaesthesia, the foetus receiving the anaesthetic via placental transfer (Bergman *et al.*, 1995). There is no report of subsequent analgesia being offered to the foetus, although presumably pain must still be present from the fresh operation site.

If it is the right of the foetus to be free from pain, it would seem that unless some method can be found to administer a peri- and post-operative analgesic regime, this right is not being respected. Increasingly, charities and organisations, such as the Women and Children's Welfare Fund, and Consumers for Ethics in Research (CERES) are taking an interest in the field of pre- and post-natal medicine, both by supporting research into foetal and infant stress, and by representing the interests of the parents (Appendix 4).

The rights of animals

When considering the ethics of research into foetal and infant pain relief, it should be remembered that frequently such research involves experimentation with animals, which for many caregivers may be a source of stress and self-questioning. This is not the place for the discussion of such a controversial subject: suffice it to say that the undoubted suffering of animals used in pain research has to be weighed against the undoubted suffering of newborn babies if pain is not treated.

Education and research go hand in hand; the more we learn, the more we discover how much we need to know. Research is needed to show how life-saving surgery may be performed on foetuses without the infliction of pain. Research is also needed to examine the long-term outcome of very preterm babies who have spent weeks on ventilators: neonatal intensive care is a relatively new science, and these babies are still children. Research may show us the effects of pain caused by medical intervention: education will teach us how to avoid inflicting it in the first place.

Chapter 11
Dying with Dignity

Death is a rite of passage and mourning is a passage from disbelief to acceptance; and since nobody lives for ever, we all at some time or other follow the process of mourning.

On the way to acceptance of death, the mourner passes through the stages of anger, apathy and grief, and if he fails to pass through these stages, he may remain in a state of *pathogenic grief*. This shows itself in physical disorders such as sleeplessness and loss of appetite, a pre-occupation with the image of the deceased, guilt, hostility and avoidance of others, and changes in usual patterns of conduct (Klaus & Kennell, 1976). *Acute grief* has been described as a sensation of bodily stress coming in waves. There is a feeling of tightness in the throat, choking and shortness of breath; there is a need to sigh accompanied by exhaustion and lack of strength, an empty and lonely feeling, a sense of unreality, and a feeling of emotional distance from other people (Lindemann, 1944). A full expression of emotional reactions in a grieving person is necessary for the optimal resolution of mourning. But at the loss of a newborn baby the mother has great difficulty in following this process, for reasons discussed below.

The parents

In the postnatal period, mother and baby still perceive themselves as one person; if the baby dies, it is as though part of the mother has gone, leaving a phantom limb in which the pain still lingers, incurable. The mother of the preterm infant, on the other hand, has already mourned the fantasy baby of her dreams; how can she now mourn the 'changeling' whom she has not been given time to recognise as her own?

The death of a newborn baby is an affront to the rituals of grief. What do friends and relations say to parents on such an occasion? They can sympathise with the affliction, but they can hardly share in mourning for someone they have never seen, and who, to them, has never existed. Even close family and friends may fail in sensitivity at such a time. Very often, with the intention of being kind, someone will try to comfort the mother by 'magical repair', telling her that she can 'soon have another', or that death is 'all for the best'. But the mother does not want to hear these things. She does not want to think of another baby while she is still bruised and aching for the loss of this one; nor does she believe it is all for the best. Sometimes friends and neighbours may not realise the extent of grief felt by the mother and will ask questions about the baby's death which she will feel obliged to answer. This will be particularly hard for her, as frequently mothers blame themselves for the death, however irrational that may be.

Fathers also have their special needs. Studies have shown that, although they may feel less guilty than the mothers, their guilt is compounded by a feeling that their grief is somehow inappropriate; 'society seems to expect men to be composed, rational and available as partner, protector and counselor'. One study found that: 'few (fathers) were acknowledged by society as having sustained a loss' (Kimble, 1991). Many fathers experience intense feelings of loneliness, isolation and futility (Lindemann, 1944).

Grief for the death of a baby may be complicated by the sense of futility that accompanies it – it is against the natural order of things that life should end before it has really begun (Brewin with Sparshott, 1996). The baby is a symbol of creativity, the child a symbol of potential growth, so parents lose not only the present, but the future as well (Hindmarch, 1993). It is important that both parents should be able to express their feelings, but people do not all grieve in the same way. Some may apprehend that they are expected to express emotions they do not at the moment feel, and this will increase their frustration, guilt and anger. Others may believe that it is wrong to express their grief externally, and will try to conceal their emotions at considerable cost to themselves – and to their relationship with their partner. The process of mourning varies in length between different people; one partner may become reconciled before the other, and this can cause tensions if it is not understood. Mourning may draw a couple together, particularly at first, but afterwards there are many problems that can arise if they are not completely open with each other.

Doctors and nurses

Doctors and nurses in a neonatal unit frequently feel a sense of guilt at the death of a baby. Doctors, particularly, find it hard to accept death, as for them it represents failure. Some doctors are held back from a frank discussion with the parents because of a sensitivity to their emotional reactions – the tears and the anger. This is a mistake, as many parents appreciate empathy from the doctor (Klaus & Kennell, 1976; Kohner & Henley, 1991; Brewin with Sparshott, 1996).

By helping parents through the mourning process, neonatal staff will help to resolve their own feelings of guilt and grief; this help should include listening to and learning from the parents. Practical guidelines for helping the bereaved are based on three premises:

(1) The bereaved person is helped to accept the death of a loved one by perceiving its concrete reality.
(2) Having acknowledged the external reality of the loss, the bereaved person needs to adapt himself or herself to it internally through the process of mourning.
(3) If the bereaved person fails to accomplish the mourning task, he or she will be unable to resume healthy progressive functioning (Furman, 1976).

As we have seen, it is difficult for parents to mourn a preterm baby because the child has not yet become a person to be loved in his own right. Parents should not be forced to do something they do not feel ready to do, but to make the baby 'real' for them it is important that they should see him and, preferably, touch him. One SHO helped a mother look at her stillborn child by sitting on her bed and talking to her, with the baby lying beside them, wrapped in a green cloth: 'After a while, she was able to feel first the baby's foot through the cloth, and gradually the whole body; then the baby was uncovered' (Jolly, 1975).

Breaking bad news

Bad news should be broken by someone who is well known to the parents of the baby, and who has a good relationship with them. Sometimes this can be a nurse, but usually it is a senior doctor who undertakes this role, as the parents may have many questions to ask, and there may be hard decisions to make. For such a discussion, a quiet room apart from the business of the unit should be found, and there should be no interruptions. Even if it seems banal, the offer of coffee or tea is often gratefully accepted, and can help to maintain a relaxed, unhurried atmosphere. Bad news should be given face to face, and eye-to-eye contact should be maintained. Parents and doctor should be sitting at the same level, with no impediment between them. Language used should be simple and natural, and the parents should be given time to assimilate what is being said, as at first they are likely to be too shocked to understand. For this reason, apart from offering added support to the parents, it is useful if the 'named nurse' or the nurse caring for the baby should also be present, as she can repeat later on what the doctor has said (Hindmarch, 1993; Brewin with Sparshott, 1996).

If there is a question of withdrawal of treatment, no decisions should be made in a hurry, as parents need to be given a chance to change their minds; they can be left with regrets if they are not given the opportunity to reconsider decisions made when in great anguish of mind. Disagreement between partners will also often resolve itself, if they are given time to see for themselves when the maintenance of mechanical life support is cruel.

Dying with dignity

The last service caregivers can render a baby is to allow him to die with dignity. When death is perceived as inevitable, it is customary nowadays to stop life support machinery and remove all non-essential monitoring equipment and treatment – but he should not be abandoned to pain at this time. The family should be together in a quiet place, preferably a room apart, and they should be left alone if they so wish. Nurses, particularly, often feel very close to the parents – they become attached to babies who have been ill for a long time – but the dying baby belongs to his parents and they should be left to grieve for him alone together, unless they request otherwise. To grieve and weep with the parents is acceptable, often inevitable. The death of a baby is stressful for the whole NICU, but it can be a time for a drawing together in mutual respect and support for caregivers and parents alike.

Some parents want to keep their baby with them for a time after his death, and if they have clothes of their own they may like to bath him and dress him themselves. They should be given the opportunity to have him with them in a separate room as long as they wish, and should feel free to ask to see him again later on.

Neonatal staff should at all times be sure they understand and respect differences in religion and culture; this is of particular importance when the baby is dying. A wrong move now can not only give offence, but also will be hurtful; this is not the time to make assumptions, or to try to promote one's own personal beliefs. If caregivers are ignorant as to what procedure to follow, they must be honest and ask relatives, or the parents themselves. Whatever their faith, if there is any ceremony the parents desire, this can be arranged, either with the hospital chaplain or with their own spiritual leader, and parents should be given either a record of this ceremony, or a card with a photograph which they can keep to remember the baby by. In their denial, parents will often refuse a photograph at first, but they can always be told that it will be put aside for them to collect later, and frequently this is what they do. Little booklets on death and bereavement, such as *Saying Goodbye to Your Baby* published by the Stillbirth and Neonatal Death Society (SANDS), may help them at this time (Appendix 4).

Siblings

Siblings have often been called 'the forgotten mourners' (Hindmarch, 1993); it is natural for parents to try to protect their children from the pain of grief, but children can see this as deception, and later on it may cause resentment. Children also need to grieve, and will be deeply disturbed if they feel excluded. It is important that they should be allowed to participate in mourning, even if death is too difficult a concept for them to grasp. If children are present, for instance, when bad news is broken, they may understand very little of what is said, but at least they will know that there are no secrets being kept from them (Wynnejones, 1985).

Children react to death in different ways, and the aspect death has for a child will depend on his age. From 1 to 3 years, death is seen as reversible; the dead are somehow 'less alive'. From 5 to 9 years, a child may understand that death is irreversible, but he will believe it can only happen to others. After the age of 10, death is seen as final, inevitable and associated with the cessation of bodily activities (Osterweis et al, 1984). Certain expressions should be avoided in the case of small children. To say that little brother has 'gone to sleep' may make the child fear to go to sleep himself, in case he sleeps for ever. To tell him that 'God has taken your little brother' may make him afraid that God will come for him, too (Jolly, 1975). Wynnejones suggests that it is the word 'take' that seems to cause trouble. A child might readily believe that if God can 'take' one child He could easily take another – himself.

Death is presented on film and television every day in forms that are violent and bloody; this may be a child's only notion of what happens, since films showing the (far more natural) quiet death of people who are loved are less frequently seen. To counterbalance this malign influence, there are available for children little booklets explaining death, such as Stickney's *Water Bugs and Dragonflies* (1984) and Varley's *Badger's Parting Gifts* (1985) for the very young child, or *Beyond the Ridge* by Goble (1993), based on the beliefs of the Plains Indians of North America, for all ages (see 'References' for details).

Little children often have jealous feelings towards new brothers and sisters, and sometimes death can be seen as a sort of 'magical punishment' rather than an end to life; children may in this case see themselves as responsible for the death by wishing it to happen. Parents can explain that they are crying because they are unhappy at the loss of the baby, not because they are angry with the children, and in fact they are comforted to have them nearby (Klaus & Kennell, 1976).

It is important not to forget adolescent siblings at a time of mourning, for they are at an age that is particularly vulnerable. In their efforts to comfort and explain dying to the smaller children, parents may leave adolescents to look to themselves for comfort, or may even expect them to help in caring for the little ones. Adolescents may have an adult understanding of death, but still be reluctant to accept its finality – like the ten-year-old boy who said, 'I know my father is dead, but what I cannot understand is why he doesn't come home for dinner' (Wynne-jones, 1985). This disbelief may present itself as an appearance of indifference, and a desire to go off by themselves or with friends. If the family circle is a large one, other family members may help adolescents share the burden they feel they have to carry; if not, parents should remember that adolescents are still young and dependent on them, and draw them into the circle, thanking them and encouraging them for the help and support they give.

Memories

Memories are all that remain for the parents of a baby who dies; all the warmth generated by sensitive and caring support given by doctors and nurses during the dying and death of the baby will count for nothing if subsequently the parents feel abandoned by the hospital staff (Brewin with Sparshott, 1996). Arrangements can be made for the parents to see a bereavement counsellor, who will explain all the procedures they will need to follow. A list of the many support services should also be made available to them (Appendix 4), and they can be advised to talk to someone who is close to them and whom they feel will best be able to share their feelings.

Once the first shock of grief is past, parents will often think of questions they would have liked to ask the doctor about the child's last illness. The doctor (frequently the consultant) who has been most responsible for their care is the best person to 'follow up', answering questions, giving information derived from post-mortem, or allaying anxieties as to future pregnancies (Brewin with Sparshott, 1996). Parents should be seen by the doctor one or two days after the death of their baby, and again several months later to see how they are coping. If there are signs of pathogenic mourning, it may be necessary to seek the help of a psychiatrist. Sedatives can be prescribed for those who lack sleep, but tranquillisers will only delay the mourning process by deadening the effects of grief.

All the local arrangements for burial and funeral should be explained to the parents; they may not wish to attend, but if they can do so it will help them realise that their baby was born and lived, even if only for a very short time. Parents are often comforted to see members of the NU staff at the baby's funeral, as this seems to emphasise that 'caring' is a continuing process. Many parents who do not hold a funeral, and who have no grave or memorial to visit after the baby's death, lack a focus for their grief (this frequently happens following miscarriage). As time passes they find they have a feeling of 'unfinished business', and that there has been no proper ending to their mourning. Caregivers should be aware that this feeling of something unaccomplished may bring parents back to the NU on the anniversary of the baby's death. Services of remembrance arranged annually by the hospital chaplain are often very well attended, by all faiths and denominations, and can be a wonderfully healing occasion for nurses and parents alike. Ceremonies can also be arranged many years after the bereavement, and these belated ceremonies can be a release to parents, who feel that they can now 'lay their grief to rest' (Kohner & Henley, 1991).

It is important that mothers do not try to have a 'replacement baby' before they have mourned the one who has died. Pregnancy may inhibit grief and mourning, so time should be allowed for the full process of mourning to take place (Forrest, 1983). There was a young mother who, losing her first baby at the age of ten months after a long and painful struggle, became pregnant again almost immediately, only to go through the same ordeal (against all odds) with the second. This nearly destroyed her; she saved herself only through her own tremendous strength and courage, and the support she received from her husband and family.

Mourning, then, requires a ceremony, a gathering together of family and friends; these things signify that the dead are gone, and can be consigned to memory. If parents can share their grief and draw their children into a family circle at the time of mourning, it will lessen the burden for all and strengthen the family tie. Mourning carries no shame with it, once the guilt has been dispelled. Caregivers can relieve their own feelings of guilt by the knowledge that they have preserved for the parents, by their caring at the death of a baby, an image of a child who was loved. The parents can remake their lives with the memory of this love.

Chapter 12
Going Home

Preparation

As the baby improves in health and grows, the neonatal staff will be less preoccupied with him. Parents sometimes bitterly resent the diminution of attention that convalescence brings. They still have worries about their baby; doctors should listen to them, and examine their baby from time to time!

Now that he is no longer such a cause for anxiety, one of the ways parents can find help in discharging their feelings of anger, boredom and frustration at the daily trek to and from hospital, is by participation in a self-help group. Parents can meet with each other to discuss their problems, and arrange for guest speakers and the showing of films, slides and other aids to understanding the developmental and medical needs of preterm infants. This freedom to express themselves and the opportunity to learn with others can improve the ability of parents to relate to their babies, and to provide them with appropriate stimulation.

Provision is made in many hospitals for the mother to keep the baby beside her if he is not seriously ill or needing special care. Low dependency babies are nursed in incubators by their mothers' bedside in Transitional Care Units, where mothers can be supervised by midwives who have experience in neonatal care. Transitional care can be provided in special wards, or in Mother-and-Baby rooms attached to the NU, or sometimes in special care nurseries attached to post-natal wards. This system gives tremendous satisfaction to mothers who, no longer separated from their babies, quickly become proficient and confident in handling them, and are more successful at breast feeding.

Many NUs have rooms or flats where parents stay overnight at need. It is advisable for the mother at least, if not both parents, to spend several nights in the unit with her baby before she takes him home (especially if he is her first) as he may be unsettled and she is likely to be nervous the first night. The parents look after the baby on their own, the nurses only acting as baby-sitters if they wish to go out.

Questions should not be left outstanding to worry the family when the baby is already home. Procedures to be taught, such as administration of medicines or gastric tube feeding, should be understood, accepted and practised by the parents well in advance, so that they feel perfectly confident in their ability. This is particularly important if the technique they are asked to practise is complex, as in the suctioning of nasal passages or the administration of low-flow oxygen; and last minute teaching of such skills as reanimation will leave them feeling insecure. If they are uncertain they may panic, and panic the baby too.

Some NUs provide parent teaching rooms where parents are shown demonstrations of routine caring procedures, such as bathing the baby, preparation of formula feeds, and sterilising equipment. These procedures may appear easy to nursing staff, but everything unknown, no matter how simple, will worry new parents. The room should be comfortably furnished, and include teaching materials, visual aids and the equipment needed for such demonstrations. A notice board for parents in this room or their sitting room can give them information on what the baby will need at home, support groups and other useful addresses. Baby magazines, articles on knitting patterns and baby-food recipes can also be made available, which besides being useful will help parents relax and feel that life is becoming 'normal'. A special 'library' of books and videos on massage and general baby care will also be appreciated, by staff as well as parents.

Home

Responsibility for the well-being of the baby and his family does not end at the NU nursery door. Nearly all parents are apprehensive as well as delighted when the time comes to say goodbye. This abrupt parting can be made less brutal by the arrangement of regular reunions for 'old' babies, and coffee mornings and tea parties for parents and siblings. Such reunions are usually enjoyed by families and staff alike.

Expert support after discharge is imperative, particularly if the baby has returned home still dependent on oxygen. Some Health Authorities employ neonatal nurses who visit the family daily in the home; ideally, the 'premature baby' or 'prem' sisters are also trained midwives, and are qualified to give advice to the mothers on obstetric problems. When both parents and 'prem' sister feel confident that her visits are no longer necessary, she can relinquish the care of mother and baby to the health visitor, who should already have visited the mother in hospital. Apart from these daily visits, which can be spaced more widely as time goes on, there are special follow-up clinics at the hospital where the baby will be seen by the consultant paediatrician who has been responsible for his care, or by one of the paediatricians on the team. If social or financial problems occur in the meantime, the 'prem' sister or health visitor can, if the parents wish, contact the social worker.

Apart from social or economic difficulties, when the parents finally get their baby home they are going to be faced 24 hours by a 'personality'. The mother will feel good with a 'cuddly' baby who snuggles into her shoulder, who ceases to cry when comforted, who looks into her eyes. This reciprocity is a kind of 'play' between them which gains meaning as mother and baby come to understand each other. The formation of a relationship such as this is sometimes difficult with a baby discharged after a long period of hospital care, because in hospital he has not learnt the rules of the game.

NICU babies can present personality problems, sometimes being too active and irritable, sometimes too inert and slow to respond; parents find it difficult to cope with such extremes in behaviour. The baby with disturbed sleep patterns will keep his parents awake and cause tension. The hyperactive and temperamental baby will be difficult to soothe and quick to fly into a tantrum. On the other hand, an immature or neuro-logically impaired baby is likely to be limp, inert and reluctant to respond to his mother's attempts to stimulate him, no matter how she exerts herself to do so; this she may perceive as rejection.

Parents can be helped to understand the individual personalities of their babies and learn how to cope with them by participating in the performance of the NBAS and listening to the examiner explain what he is doing, and what the responses mean. In one study, teenaged dis-advantaged mothers were encouraged to watch caregivers give NBAS examinations to their preterm infants, and were then asked to fill out a weekly rating scale, similar to the NBAS ratings. Apparently the most popular item with the girls was engaging the baby's attention with a red ball (Widmayer & Field, 1980). These young girls later became successful mothers.

Brazelton recognises variability in the temperament of babies; whether they be average, quiet or active, he encourages parents to adjust to the differences in their babies, and see them as unique (Brazelton, 1983).

Colic

The subject of colic is relevant here because it has been suggested that colicky babies are more susceptible to child abuse: 'both the aversive sound of the cry and the helplessness that parents may feel when faced by the colicky baby have been suggested as the mechanisms linking colic and abuse' (McGrath & Unruh, 1987). Infants have the highest incidence of colic when their mothers are anxious or tense in handling them, and this is likely to be improved by both treatment of the mother's anxiety and amelioration of the family situation (Prugh *et al.*, 1983). Nervousness in the parent is nearly always transmitted to the baby; it is also possible that the circle is a vicious one, and that the nervousness and tension the mother feels on hearing her baby cry may be transmitted to him, and exacerbate the condition.

The colicky baby screams and will not be comforted; this seems to happen mostly in the evening, when parents are hoping to relax. Carrying the baby prone across the arms, with a hand supporting the abdomen, may ease his discomfort (Walker, 1995) (Fig. 12.1). Some

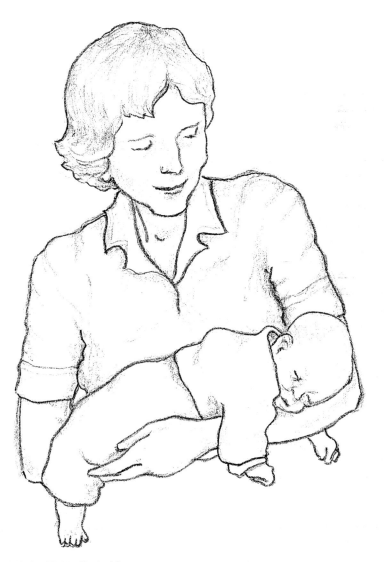

Fig. 12.1 The colic hold.

studies have shown that colicky babies can be soothed by domestic sounds such as a vacuum cleaner or the washing machine (McGrath & Unruh, 1987). For the parent to be forced to clean the carpets every time the baby cries seems a depressing form of treatment, especially if the baby becomes habituated to the sound and does not want it to stop!

Parents need to be shown how to cope with a crying baby, of which the baby with colic is an irritating example. No baby is as uncuddly as the baby with colic! Parents can only be encouraged by the fact that colic will eventually disappear spontaneously.

Enjoy!

With all these difficulties to surmount, it is surprising that a mother ever comes to terms with her preterm or sick baby, and that he ever manages to ingratiate himself into the bosom of his family – but she does and he does. For this successful outcome to come about, sensitive support for the parents is needed from the beginning.

Winnicott shows the mother how the pleasure she experiences with her baby is important for both of them:

> 'I know you will enjoy the signs that gradually appear that the baby is a person, and that you are recognized as a person by the baby ... If you are there enjoying it all, it is like the sun coming out, for the baby. The mother's pleasure has to be there or else the whole procedure is dead, useless and mechanical.' (Winnicott, 1957)

Conclusion
The All-embracing Harmony

'The aim of all human striving is to establish – or, probably, re-establish – an all-embracing harmony with one's environment, to be able to love in peace.' (Balint, 1968)

Neonatology is both a new and an old science. As long ago as the 4th century BC Plato said:

'The first step, as you know, is always what matters most, particularly when we are dealing with those who are young and tender. That is the time when they are taking shape and when any impression we choose to make leaves a permanent mark.'

It is not only the baby who experiences discomfort in the NU. Parents and nurses are also affected by their perception of the baby as either offspring or patient, and the need to justify the traumatic procedures inflicted on him in the name of caregiving. Parents feel that they can only look on while doctors and nurses assault their babies; doctors and nurses are worried about the possible consequences of their actions, and are frustrated that they cannot do more to avoid them.

'Making a home' on the NU which will help to assuage pain and distress means the creation of a holding environment for all concerned – an ambience of mutual dependence and confidence. All parents are not sensible and loving, all nurses are not selfless and kind, all doctors are not clever and confident, but it is best to start from this premise – much of the time it will be true.

The babies who pass the first part of their lives in the NICU are nourished by their caregivers; now we must learn to cherish them as well. Throughout this book we have seen the ways caregivers and researchers have sought to improve the lot of newborn babies, not always agreeing with each other on how this should be done; some of you will yourselves disagree with points made, because you have had different experiences. But we will all agree on one point; every baby is unique – individuals every one! We cannot know what the future holds for our babies, or what sort of people they are going to be. Certainly the

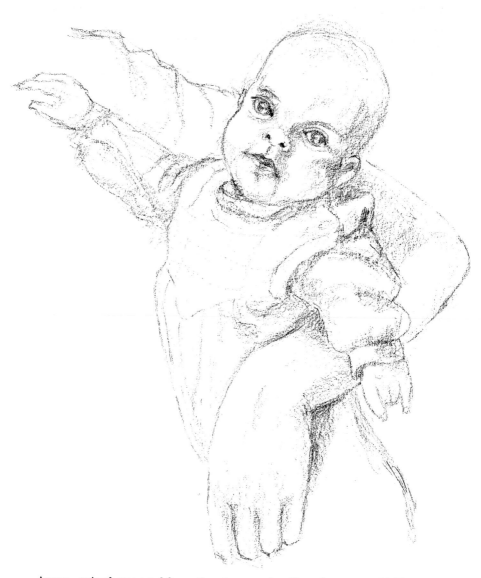

Aaron – going home aged 6 months, strong and resilient (compare with Fig. 5.5).

babies who survive show amazing strength and resilience; nor, when they return to visit, do they seem to have distressing memories of their medical and nursing caregivers – on the contrary, frequently we are greeted with smiles.

Babies must be given their chance of survival. If we create for them the most favourable environment possible, if we study to understand them better, and if we continue to seek ways to protect them from pain, the future of these babies must take care of itself. After all, whether the baby is born 'too soon or too small', life will present him with his share of pain and terror, joy and rapture. He may arrive at a mellow old age, battered but triumphant, wondering how quickly the years have passed him by; he may founder somewhere along the road, due possibly to damage caused by the care he received at the beginning. The preterm baby may grow to be the pride of his parents' lives – or he may be the bane of their existence – but at least he is alive to choose which it will be!

Appendix 1
Behavioural Responses of the Newborn Infant to Pain

(a) Facial expression

Neonatal Facial Coding System (NFCS) (Grunau & Craig, 1987)

- Brow bulge   bulging, creasing and vertical furrows above and between brows.
- Eye-squeeze   squeezing or bulging of eyelids.
- Naso-labial furrow   pulling upwards and deepening of furrow between nostril wings and lip corners.
- Open/stretched mouth   wide open mouth, tautness of lip corners, downward pull on jaw and horizontal pull at corners of mouth.
- Lip purse   as if 'oo' is being pronounced.
- Taut tongue   raised, cupped tongue with sharp raised edges.
- Chin quiver   high frequency up–down motion of the lower jaw.

Other observed response

- Frantic sucking (Debillon, 1992).

(b) Body movement

Infant Body Coding System (IBCS) (Craig *et al.*, 1993)

Variable name	Description
Hand/foot movements	include flexion, extension or rotation at the wrist, and spreading, grasping or twitching of the fingers. Foot movements include flexion, extension or rotation at the ankle, and spreading, twitching or flaring of the toes.

Variable name	Description
Arm movements	include well-modulated, jerky or limited movements, and well-modulated movements that involve a transition from flexion to extension, or vice versa, or ad/abduction accomplished smoothly without jerkiness. In *well-modulated* movements the arc of motion appears controlled and unrestricted, with one movement frequently moving into the next. *Jerky* movements involve sudden abrupt oscillation from extension to flexion, or vice versa, dramatic startles and twitches, or movements that are restricted by something in their path. *Limited* movements include twisting or writhing of the limbs close to the body.
Leg movements	include well-modulated, jerky and/or limited movements (see above for descriptions).
Head movements	include lateral activity, head turn and neck flexion or extension.
Torso movements	include resisting, arching, twisting or writhing in the torso.
Other observed responses	
Moro reflex	'startle' reflex with arms jerked back, then returned to midline with fingers flared (but this reaction is predominantly due to fear of loss of support).
Extension	complete extension and rigidity of all extremities (Debillon, 1992).
Withdrawal	withdrawal of one or both limbs from source of injury.
Side-swiping	side-swiping with unaffected limb (Dale, 1986).

(c) Extreme pain (Gauvain-Piquard, 1989b; Sparshott, 1989a)

- Antalgic position at rest – an unnatural position adopted by the body as a defence against pain.
- Axial stiffening.
- Head thrown back.
- Abnormal position of limbs.
- No reponse to consoling techniques.

(d) Long lasting pain (Gauvain-Piquard, 1989b; Sparshott, 1989a)

- No crying.
- Reduced spontaneous motor activity.
- Diminished communication with the outside world – minimal response to stimuli – lack of response to caregiver.
- Diminished alertness.
- Hostility – eye avoidance – fixed or staring gaze (expression of 'frozen watchfulness').

Appendix 2
Distress Scale for Ventilated Newborn Infants (DSVNI)

Table 1 DSVNI score sheet.

Name: Date: Time: Hospital number:

Gestation: Age: Birth weight:

Main diagnosis:

Type of ventilation: Duration of ventilation:

Analgesia or local anaesthetic: Dose:

Time since last given:

Bolus/infusion:

Traumatic procedure: No. of attempts:

Duration of procedure:

Score	Baseline	During procedure	After procedure At 3 mins	At 1 hr	Time taken to return to baseline
Facial expression					
Body movement					
Colour					
Heart rate*					
Blood pressure*					
Oxygen saturation*					
Temperature – skin* – toe*					
Total					

Code for invasive procedures:

CD	Chest drain insertion	LP	Lumbar puncture
INT	Intubation	VP	Venepuncture
ETS	Endotracheal suctioning	AS	Arterial stab
OPS	Oropharangeal suctioning	HL	Heel-lance
CPAP	Continuous positive airways pressure		Other

*To avoid more disturbance to the baby, these observations need only be made if monitoring equipment is already in place.

(From Sparshott, 1996.)

Table 2   DSVNI scoring system.

Behavioural score

Facial expression

0 'relaxed'   smooth muscled; relaxed expression; either in deep sleep or quietly alert

1 'anxious'   anxious expression; frown; REM behind closed lids; wandering gaze; eyes narrowed; lips parted; pursed lips as if 'oo' is being pronounced

2 'anguished'   anguished expression/crumpled face; brow bulge; eye-squeeze; naso-labial furrow pronounced; square-stretched mouth; cupped tongue; 'silent cry'

3 'inert'   (only during or immediately following traumatic procedure) no response to trauma; no crying; rigidity; gaze avoidance; fixed/staring gaze; apathy; diminished alertness

Body movement

0 'relaxed'   relaxed trunk and limbs; body in tucked position; hands in cupped position or willing to grasp a finger

1 'restless'   Moro reflex; startles; jerky or unco-ordinated movement of limbs; flexion/extension of limbs; attempt to withdraw limb from site of injury

2 'exaggerated'   abnormal position of limbs; limb/neck extension; splaying of fingers and/or toes; flailing or thrashing of limbs; arching back; side-swiping/guarding site of injury

3 'inert'   (only during or immediately following traumatic procedure) no response to trauma; inertia; limpness/rigidity; immobility

Colour

0   normal skin colour (depending on skin type)
1   redness; congestion
2   pallor; mottling; grey

Physiological changes

Physiological changes are not scored, but read directly from the monitors. Changes indicative of stress read from baseline, are:

Heart rate   increase; decrease; bradycardia frequent in fragile infants

Blood pressure   increase

Oxygenation   commonly decrease; occasionally increase due to crying and consequent increased intracranial pressure

Temperature differential   widening gap in core and peripheral temperature; decrease in peripheral temperature

(From Sparshott, 1996.)

Table 3 Operational definitions.

Behavioural score	0	1	2	3
Facial expression	*'Relaxed'* Smooth muscled; unlined relaxed expression; deep sleep/quiet alert state	*'Anxious'* Anxious expression; frown; REM; wandering gaze/eyes narrowed; lips parted/pursed	*'Anguished'* Anguished expression/crumpled face; brow bulge; eye-squeeze; naso-labial furrow; square/stretched mouth; cupped tongue; 'silent cry'	*'Inert'* (no response to trauma) No crying; gaze avoidance; fixed/staring gaze; rigidity; diminished alertness
	Deep sleep state *Quiet alert state*	*Eyes tightly closed; pursed lips* *Eyes narrowed/ wandering gaze; lips pursed/slightly parted*	*Silent cry* *Cupped tongue*	*Gaze avoidance* *Fixed/staring gaze*
Body movement	*'Relaxed'* Relaxed trunk and limbs; tucked position; cupped hands/finger grasp	*'Restless'* Moro reflex; startles; jerky; unco-ordinated movements; limb flexion/extension; limb withdrawal	*'Exaggerated'* Limb/neck extension; finger/toe splay; flailing; thrashing of limbs; arching back; side-swiping; guarding	*'Inert'* (no response to trauma) Inertia; immobility; limpness/rigidity
	Relaxed trunk and limbs *Tucked position*	*Limb withdrawal*	*'Exaggerated' neck extension; flailing; arching back* *'Exaggerated' limb extension; finger/toe splay*	*Rigidity*
Colour	Normal skin colour according to type	Redness; congestion	Pallor; mottling; grey	Baseline colour; pallor, mottling, grey

(From Sparshott, 1996.)

Assessment of behavioural score

0   'relaxed – infant comfortable, not distressed.

1–2   some transitory distress caused; returns immediately to 'relaxed'.

3–4   transitory distress, likely to respond to consolation.

5   infant experiences pain; if no response to consolation, may require analgesia.

6   'anguished' and 'exaggerated' – infant experiencing acute pain; is unlikely to respond to consolation, will probably benefit from analgesia.

6–8   'inert – (no reponse to traumatic procedure) infant is habituated to pain; will not respond to consolation; systematic pain control by analgesia should be considered.

Appendix 3
Infant Stimulation Care Plan

	Goals	Nursing intervention	Rationale
Visual	Maintains eye-to-eye contact.	Initiate eye-to-eye contact.	Fosters identification and attachment.
	Focuses for at least 3 seconds. Tracks visual tool at least 15 degrees laterally and to midline.	Show infant his/her favourite black-and-white pattern for three 10 second intervals during two alert periods per day. Alternate holding the pattern still and moving it across infant's visual field.	Increases concentration and ability to follow.
	Focuses for at least 5 seconds. Begins reaching behaviour (extending) (fingers and toes).	Present mobile for 1–2 minutes at least b.i.d.	Infants focus more readily on moving objects
Tactile	Maintains regular respiratory effort. Periods of disruptive motor activity and alert inactivity cease.	Provide slow (12 strokes/minute) skin-to-skin stroking in head-to-toe direction for 15 minutes/day.	Skin-to-skin stroking provides warmth. Head-to-toe stroking enhances myelination
	Exhibits decreased muscle activity, even respirations. Heart rate slows by 8 beats/minute.	Provide an alternative stimulus (sheepskin, deep pile velvet) for 10 minutes at least daily.	Prevents habituation and stimulates haptic nerves for motor growth.
Auditory	Head turns to locate sound. Assumes flexed position. Becomes more alert.	Play tape of parents' voices for 2–3 minutes q.i.d. during alert inactivity.	Fosters attachment and recognition of parents. Stimulates left hemisphere of brain.
	Assumes quiescence or arousal. Demonstrates snuggling behaviour.	Play classical music (music box or recording) for 5 minutes q.i.d.	Stimulates right hemisphere. Helps develop fine sense tonality
	Orients to sound by turning head. Alerts to his/her name.	Call infant by name at each interaction.	Enhances recognition of self. Captures attention.
	Attempts vocalisation and imitation. Responds to voice with rhythmic movements.	Speak with various inflections. Alternate adult speech and baby talk.	Inflection holds attention longer than base. Adult speech increases understanding Baby talk facilitates language acquisition.

Category			
Vestibular	Maintains even, deep respirations with less apnoea. Gains weight steadily.	Use waterbed at 10 oscillations/minute and 3 waves/oscillation. Alternate 10 minutes' oscillation with rest periods.	Helps regulate respiratory function. Rest periods prevent habituation to oscillation.
	Assumes flexion, visual attentiveness or quiescence.	Rock in chair, front to back, 16 rocks/minute.	Encourages memory development.
	Head lag decreases.	Lift head to upright position, tip to right and then to left, stopping at midline.	Encourages righting reflex which accelerates myelination.
	Grasp reflex attenuated.	Close infant's fist around a cloth toy (stuffed ball or cylinder).	Enhances grasp reflex. Promotes self-stimulation of bringing object within visual field.
	Offers more powerful and purposeful resistance.	Give passive exercise to knee and hip by alternatively flexing and extending hip and knee before each feeding.	Exercise increases myelination and muscle growth and control. Provides enjoyable interaction.
Olfactory	Alert, with slight flexive movements of extremities.	Pass open breast milk container under nose t.i.d.	Initiates olfactory movements. Helps identify mother by smell.
		Pass sweet smell (cherry juice, nutmeg, cinnamon, strawberry extract) under nose.	Encourages association of sweet smells with caregiver. Stimulates some of the 3000 receptors in the nose.
Gustatory	Increases self-regulated sucking and saliva production.	Place infant's hand or pacifier in his/her mouth when sucking motions are observed or during gavage feedings.	Hand-in-mouth is active stimulation, which has a greater effect than passive. Saliva may accelerate growth and development and help prevent necrotising enterocolitis.
	Increases saliva production and speed of digestion.	Place 2 drops of milk in mouth with each tube feeding.	Acquaints infant with taste of milk. Improves digestion.

(From Chaze & Ludington-Hoe (1984) Sensory Stimulation in the NICU. *American Journal of Nursing*, **84**, No. 1, January, 70/71, with permission.)

Appendix 4
Useful Addresses

Assessment of Preterm Infant Behavior (APIB)

Heidelise Als, PhD
Director
J. Layla Faxon, MBA
Contact
National APIB Training Center
Enders Pediatric Research Laboratories
Room EN-029
The Children's Hospital
320 Longwood Avenue
Boston
MA 02115
Tel: 617 355 8249
Fax: 617 355 7230

Counselling

British Association for Counselling
1 Regent Place
Rugby
Warwickshire CV21 2PJ
Tel: (01788) 578 328 (information line)

The national voice on issues related to counselling. Lists of counsellors and counselling agencies in local areas may be obtained by sending an A4 stamped addressed envelope to the above address.

Royal College of Nursing Counselling and Advisory Service
8–10 Crown Hill
Croydon
Surrey CR0 1RZ
Tel: (0345) 697 064 (RCN members' line)
Tel: (0181) 667 9787
Fax: (0181) 681 5030

Offers a free short-term and confidential service to RCN members on a range of personal or work related issues.

Ethics

Consumers for Ethics in Research (CERES)
PO Box 1365
London N16 0BW

A forum that holds meetings and publishes reports especially about health service users' views about medical research.

Help-lines for parents and families

Action for Sick Children
29–31 Euston Road
London NW1 2SD
Tel: (0171) 833 2041

Campaigns for improvements in standard and quality of child health care in hospital, at home and in the community

Baby Live Support System (BLISS) (also Blisslink/Nippers)
17–21 Emerald Street
London WC1N 3QL
Tel: (0171) 831 9393
Freecall no. (0500) 151 617
Fax: (0171) 404 3811

Leading national charity which purchases essential lifesaving equipment for NUs, sponsors nurse training and offers support and information to parents with babies who need specialist care at birth.

The Compassionate Friends
53 North Street
Bristol BS3 1EN
Tel: (0117) 953 9639
Fax: (0117) 966 5202

A nationwide organisation of bereaved parents offering friendship and understanding to other bereaved parents, with links around the world.

Contact a Family
170 Tottenham Court Road
London W1P 0HA
Tel: (0171) 383 3555
Fax: (0171) 383 0259

Gives advice/support and information to families caring for children with any form of disability or special need. Supports families of preterm and sick infants.

Stillbirth and Neonatal Death Society (SANDS)
28 Portland Place
London W1N 4DE
Tel: (0171) 436 5881

Offers support to bereaved parents, their families, friends and the health professionals involved in their care. Local groups, publications and information.

Support In Bereavement for Brothers and Sisters
PO Box 295
York YO2 5YP

SIBBS is run by bereaved siblings for bereaved siblings.

Massage

D. Adamson-Macedo, PhD (TAC-TIC)
School of Health Sciences
62–68 Lichfield Street
Wolverhampton WV1 1SB
Tel: (01902) 28525 321 000

Peter Walker
PO Box 8293
London W9 2WZ

Book and video – addresses for classes in baby massage.

Neonatal Behavioral Assessment Scale (NBAS)

J. Kevin Nugent, PhD
Director
BNBAS Training
The Brazelton Center for Infants and Parents
1295 Boylston Street
Boston
MA 02215
Tel: 617 355 4959
Fax: 617 859 7215

Neonatal Individualized Developmental Care and Assessment Program (NIDCAP)

Heidelise Als, PhD
Director
J. Layla Faxon, MBA
Contact
National NIDCAP Training Center
Enders Pediatric Research Laboratories
Room EN-029
The Children's Hospital
320 Longwood Avenue
Boston
MA 02115
Tel: 617 355 8249
Fax: 617 355 7230

Pain

International Association for the Study of Pain (IASP)
909 NE 43rd Street
Suite 305
Seattle
WA 98105
Tel: 206 547 6409
Fax: 206 547 1703

For information on education in pain management, international conferences and the journal *Pain*. Membership for health professionals.

Research

Women and Children's Welfare Fund
Administrator, Carol Banfield
Tower Office, Jedburgh, Roxburghshire TD8 6NX
Tel: (01273) 309 947

To ensure the welfare of women and children through expert accurate counselling and scrupulous medical care, including supporting research into pre- and post-natal experience.

Therapcutic Touch (TT)

Jean Sayre-Adams RN, MA
Senior Tutor
The Didsbury Trust
Sherborne Cottage
Litton
Nr. Bath
Avon BA3 4PS
Tel: (01761) 241 640

Information on training courses for therapeutic touch.

References

Abajian, J.C. & Sethna, N.F. (1993) Regional and topical anaesthesia. In: *Pain in Neonates*. Pain Research and Clinical Management, Vol. 5 (eds J.K.S. Anand & P.J. McGrath). Elsevier, Amsterdam.

Adamson-Macedo, E.N. & Attree, J.L.A. (1994) TAC-TIC therapy: the importance of systematic stroking. *British Journal of Midwifery*, **2**(6), 264–9.

Affonso, D., Bosque, E., Wahlberg, V. & Brady, J.P. (1993) Reconciliation and healing for mothers through skin-to-skin contact provided in an American tertiary level intensive care nursery. *Neonatal Network*, **12**(3), 25–32.

Als, H., Lester, B.M., Tronick, E.Z. & Brazelton, T.B. (1982) Manual for the Assessment of Preterm Infant Behavior (APIB). In: *Theory and Research in Behavioral Pediatrics*, Vol. 1 (eds H.E. Fitzgerald, B.M. Lester & M. Yogman). Plenum Press, New York.

Als, H. (1986) A synactive model of neonatal behavioral organization: framework for the assessment of neurobehavioral development in the premature infant and support of infants and parents in the neonatal intensive care environment. *Physical and Occupational Therapy in Pediatrics*, **6**, 3–53.

Als, H., Lawhon, G., Brown, E., Gibes, R., Duffy, F.H., McAnulty, G. & Blickman, J.G. (1986) Individualized behavioral and environmental care for the very low birth weight preterm infant at high risk for bronchopulmonary dysplasia: neonatal intensive care unit and developmental outcome. *Pediatrics*, **78**, 1123–32.

'Althea' (1986) *Special Care Babies*. Dinosaur Publications, London.

Amiel-Tison, C. & Grenier, A. (1986) *Neurological Assessment During the First Year of Life*. Oxford University Press, New York.

Anand, J.K.S. (1986) Hormonal and metabolic functions of neonates and infants undergoing surgery. *Current Opinion in Cardiology*, **1**, 681–9.

Anand, J.K.S. (1993) The applied physiology of pain. In: *Pain in Neonates*. Pain Research and Clinical Management, Vol. 5 (eds J.K.S. Anand & P.J. McGrath). Elsevier, Amsterdam.

Anand, J.K.S. & Hickey, P.R. (1987) Pain and its effects in the newborn neonate and fetus. *The New England Journal of Medicine*, **317**(21), 1321–9.

Anand, J.K.S., Sippell, W.G. & Aynsley-Green, A. (1987) Randomised trial of fentanyl anaesthesia in preterm babies undergoing surgery: effects on the stress response. *Lancet*, 31 January, 243–7.

Anand, J.K.S., Shapiro, B.S. & Berde, C.B. (1993) Pharmacotherapy and systemic analgesics. In: *Pain in Neonates*. Pain Research and Clinical Management, Vol. 5 (eds J.K.S. Anand & P.J. McGrath). Elsevier, Amsterdam.

Anders, T.F., & Chalemian, R.J. (1974) The effects of circumcision on sleep–awake states in human neonates. *Psychosomatic Medicine*, **36**, 174–9.

Anderson, L.J.A. & Anderson, J.M. (1988) Hand splinting for infants in the intensive care and special care nurseries. *The American Journal of Occupational Therapy*, **42**(4), 222–6.

Andrews, K. & Wills, B. (1992) A systematic approach can reduce side effects: A protocol for pain relief in neonates. *Professional Nurse*, **7**(8), 528–32.

Anzieu, D. (1974) L'enveloppe sonore du soi. In: *Le Moi-Peau*, p. 172. Editions Dunod, Paris.

Atkinson, J. & Braddick, O. (1982) Sensory and perceptual capacities of the neonate. In: *Psychobiology of the Human Newborn* (ed P.I. Stratton). John Wiley, London.

Attia, J., Amiel-Tison, C., Mayer, M.N., Schnider, D.M. & Barrier, G. (1987) Measurement of postoperative pain and narcotic administration in infants using a new scoring system. *Anesthesiology*, **67**(3A), A532.

Auckett, A.D. (1981) *Baby Massage: The Magic of the Loving Touch*. Thorsons Publishers, Wellingborough.

Aynsley-Green, A. (1987) Pain, anaesthesia and babies. *Lancet*, 5 September, 543–4.

Balint, M. (1968) *The Basic Fault: Therapeutic Aspects of Regression*. Tavistock Press, London.

Barnard, K.E. (1973) The effect of stimulation on the sleep behaviour of the premature infant. *Communicating Nursing Research*, **6**(12), 12–33.

Beail, N. (1983) The psychology of fatherhood. *Bulletin of British Psychological Society*, **36**, 312–4.

Beaver, K. (1987) Premature infants' response to touch and pain: can nurses make a difference? *Neonatal Network*, **6**(3), 13–17.

Bee, H. (1985) *The Developing Child*. Harper & Row, New York.

Bell, S.G. (1994) The national pain management guideline: implications for neonatal intensive care. *Neonatal Network*, **13**(3), 9–17.

Bellig, L.L. (1989) A window on the neonate's brain. *Neonatal Network*, **7**(4), 13–20.

Bender, H. & Swan-Parente, A. (1983) Psychological and psychotherapeutic support of staff and parents in an intensive care baby unit. In: *Parent–Baby Attachment in Premature Infants* (eds J.A. Davis, M.M.P. Richards & N.R.C. Roberton). Croom Helm, Beckenham.

Berger, B. (1981) Chloé. In: *Un Enfant, prématurément*. Ouvrage collectif sous la direction de Laurent Le Vaguerese, *les Cahiers du Nouveau-né* Vol. 6. Editions Stock, Paris.

Bergman, K., Kenner, C., Hummel Levine, A. & Inturrisi, M. (1995) Fetal Therapy. *Comprehensive Neonatal Nursing* (eds C. Kenner, A. Brueggemeyer & L.P. Gunderson), pp. 887–902. W.B. Saunders Co., Philadelphia.

Bernbaum, J.C., Pereira, G.R., Watkins, J.B. & Peckham, G.J. (1983) Non-nutritive sucking during gavage feeding enhances growth and maturation in premature infants. *Pediatrics*, **71**, 41–5.

Berne, E. (1986) *A Layman's Guide to Psychiatry and Psychoanalysis*. Penguin Books, London.

Bess, F.H., Finlayson-Peek, B. & Chapman, J.J. (1979) Further observations on noise levels and infant incubators. *Pediatrics*, **63**, 100–106.

Bissenden, J.G. (1986) Ethical aspects of neonatal care. *Archives of Disease in Childhood*, **61**, 639–41.

Blackburn, S.T. & VandenBerg, K.A. (1995) Assessment and Management of neonatal neurobehavioral development. In: *Comprehensive Neonatal Nursing* (eds C. Kenner, A. Brueggemeyer & L.P. Gunderson), pp. 1095–1130. W.B. Saunders Co., Philadelphia.

Blain-Lewis, N. (1992) Comparative studies of bruising and healing after heel-stick. *Neonatal Intensive Care*, September/October, 18–23.

Blass, E.M. & Hoffmeyer, L.B. (1991) Sucrose as an analgesic for newborn infants. *Pediatrics*, **87**, 215–18.

Blennow, G., Svenningsen, N.W. & Almquist, B. (1974) Noise levels in infant incubators (adverse effects?). *Pediatrics*, **53**, 29–32.

Boelen-van der Loo, W.J.C., van der Heide, D., Kluft, O. & Huijer-Abu-Saad, H. (1989) Postsurgical pain in children, p. 30, abstract. In: *First European Conference on Pain in Children*, Maastricht, The Netherlands, 1–2 June.

Bowlby, J. (1969) *Attachment*. Pelican Books, London.

Bradley, R.M. & Stern, I.B. (1967) The development of the human taste bud during foetal period. *Journal of Anatomy*, **104**(4), 745–52.

Brazelton, T.B. (1961) Psychophysiologic reactions in the neonate. 1: The value of observation of the neonate. *Journal of Pediatrics*, **58**, 508–12.

Brazelton, T.B. (1983) *Infants and Mothers* (revised edition). Delta/Seymour Lawrence, New York.

Brazelton, T.B. (1984) Neonatal Behavioral Assessment Scale, 2nd edn. *Clinics in Developmental Medicine, Vol. 88*. Spastics International Medical Publications, London.

Brazelton, T.B. & Nugent, J.K. (1995) *Neonatal Behavioral Assessment Scale*, 3rd edn. Mac Keith Press, London.

Brazy, J.E. (1988) Effects of crying on cerebral blood volume and cytochrome aa3. *Journal of Pediatrics*, **112**(3), 457–61.

Brenig, F.A. (1982) *Infant Incubator Study*. Dissertation for the Degree of Doctor of Public Health, School of Public Health, Faculty of Medicine, Colombia University.

Brewin, T. with Sparshott, M.M. (1996) *Relating to the Relatives*. Radcliffe Medical Press, Oxford.

Brown, L. (1987) Physiological responses to cutaneous pain in neonates. *Neonatal Network*, **6**(3), 18–22.

Brykczynska, G. (1994) Ethical issues in the neonatal unit. In: *Neonatal Nursing* (eds D. Crawford & M. Morris). Chapman & Hall, London.

Burton, I.F. & Derbyshire, A.J. (1958) 'Sleeping fit' caused by excruciating pain in an infant. *Journal of Disease in Childhood*, **96**, 258–60.

Caplan, G., Mason, E. & Kaplan, D.M. (1965) Four studies in crisis in parents of prematures. *Community Mental Health Journal*, **1**, 149–61.

Carter, J. (1974) *The Maltreated Child*. Priory Press, London.

Chamberlain, D.B. (1989) Babies remember pain. *Pre-and Peri-Natal Psychology*, **3**(4), 297–310.

Chaze, B.A. & Ludington-Hoe, S.M. (1984) Sensory stimulation in the NICU. *American Journal of Nursing*, **84**, No. 1, January, 68–71.

Chiswick, M.L. & Roberton, N.C. (1987) Doctors and nurses in neonatal intensive care: towards integration. *Archives of Disease in Childhood*, 62, 653–5.

Colditz, P.B. (1991) Management of pain in the newborn infant (review article). *Journal of Pediatric Child Health*, **27**, 11–15.

Cole, J.G. & Frappier, P.A. (1985) Infant stimulation reassessed: a new approach to providing care for the preterm infant. *Journal of Obstetric, Gynocologic and Neonatal Nursing*. November/December, 471–77.

Connolly, J.A. & Cullen, J.H. (1983) Maternal stress and the origins of health status. In: *Frontiers of Infant Psychiatry* (eds. J.D. Call, E. Galensen & R.L. Tyson), pp. 273–81. Basic Books, New York.

Copp, L.A. (1985) Pain, ethics and the negotiation of values. In: *Perspectives on Pain* (ed. Copp L.A.) Churchill Livingstone, New York.

Cornick, P. (1989) A cry for help? Management of postoperative pain and discomfort in neonates. *Professional Nurse*, June, 457–9.

Craig, K.D. & Grunau, R.V.E. (1993) Neonatal pain perception and behavioral measurement. In: *Pain in Neonates*. Pain Research and Clinical Management, Vol. 5 (ed K.J.S. Anand & P.J. McGrath). Elsevier, Amsterdam.

Craig, K.D., Whitfield, M.F., Grunau, R.V.E., Linton, J. & Hadjistavropoulos, H.D. (1993) Pain and the preterm neonate: behavioral and physiological indices. *Pain*, **52**, 287–99.

Cramer, B. (1976) A mother's reaction to the birth of a premature baby. In: *Maternal–Infant Bonding* (eds M. Klaus & J.H. Kennell). C.V. Mosby, St Louis.

Crawford, D. (1994) Infant neurology. In: *Neonatal Nursing* (eds D. Crawford & M. Morris). Chapman & Hall, London.

Cunningham, N. *et al.* (1987) Infant carrying, breast feeding and mother–infant relations. *Lancet*, 14 February.

Cunningham, N. (1993) Moral and ethical issues in clinical practice. In: *Pain in Neonates*. Pain Research and Clinical Management, Vol. 5 (eds K.J.S. Anand & P.J. McGrath). Elsevier, Amsterdam.

Dale, J.C. (1986) A multidimensional study of infants' responses to painful stimuli. *Pediatric Nursing*, **12**(1), 27–31.

d'Apolito, K. (1984) The neonate's response to pain. *Maternal–Child Nursing*, **6**, 28–32.

de Bel, C. (1989) Pain in the pediatric department, p. 27, abstract. In: *First European Conference on Pain in Children*, Maastricht, The Netherlands, 1–2 June.

Debillon, T. (1992) Controle de la douleur en néonatologie. In: *Fourth International Symposium* of B.I.S.P.I.C., Centre Hospitalo–Universitaire, Bicêtre, Paris, 26 September, 84–91.

De Caspar, A.J. & Fifer, W.P. (1980) Of human bonding: newborns prefer their mothers' voices. *Science*, **208**, 1174–6.

Dobbs-Zeller, B., Parratte, D. & Poletti, R. (1984) *Reflexologie pour les Professionels de la Santé*. Editions Sophia, Geneva.

Dollison, E.J. & Beckstrand, J. (1995) Adhesive tape vs Pectin-based barrier use in preterm infants. *Neonatal Network*, **14**(4), 35–9.

Dowie, R. (1989) *Patterns of medical staffing*. Interim report, British Postgraduate Medical Federation, London.

Dreyfus-Brisac, C. (1983) Organisation of sleep in prematures: implications for care giving. In: *Frontiers of Infant Psychiatry* (eds J.D. Call, E. Galenson & R.L. Tyson). Basic Books, New York.

Drillien, C.M. (1964) *The Growth and Development of the Prematurely Born Infant*. Churchill Livingstone, Edinburgh.

Edwards, S. (1995) Phototherapy and the neonate: providing safe and effective nursing care for jaundiced infants. *Journal of Neonatal Nursing*, **1**(5), 9–12.

Elander, G. (1989) Post-operative pain relief in infancy, p. 29, abstract. In: *First International Conference on Pain in Children*, Maastricht, The Netherlands, 1–2 June.

Emde, R., Harmon, R. Metcalf, D., Koenig, K. & Wagonfeld, S. (1971) Stress and neonatal sleep. *Psychosomatic Medicine*, **33**, 491–7.

Emery, M.L. (1996) Periventricular/intraventricular haemorrhage in the preterm infant. *Journal of Neonatal Nursing*, **2**(1), 16–18.

Engel, R. (1964) Electroencephalographic responses to photic stimulation, and the correlation with maturation. *Annals of the New York Academy of Science*, **117**, 407–12.

Erikson, E. (1963) *Childhood and Society*, pp. 247–51. W.W. Norton, New York.

Evans, N.J. & Rutter, N. (1986) Reduction of skin damage from transcutaneous oxygen electrode using a spray-on dressing. *Archives of Disease in Childhood*, **61**, 881–4.

Field, T., Hallock, N., Ting, G. *et al.* (1978) A first year follow-up of high risk infants: formulating a cumulative high risk index. *Child Development*, **49**, 119–31.

Field, T. (1982) Differential affective displays of high-risk infants during early interaction. In: *Emotion and Interaction: Normal and High Risk Infants* (eds T. Field & A. Fogel). Erlbaum, Hillsdale, New Jersey.

Field, T. (1992) Interventions in early infancy. *Infant Mental Health Journal*, **13**(4), 329–36.

Fitzgerald, M., Millard, C. & McIntosh, N. (1989) Cutaneous hypersensitivity following tissue damage in newborn infants and its reversal with topical anaesthesia. *Pain*, **39**, 31–6.

Flandermeyer, A.A. (1995) The drug exposed neonate. In: *Comprehensive Neonatal Nursing* (eds C. Kenner, A. Brueggemeyr & L.P. Gunderson), pp. 997–1033. W.B. Saunders, Philadelphia.

Fletcher, A. (1979) Working in a neonatal intensive care unit. Paper presented to a meeting of the Scientific Applied Section. Tavistock Clinic, London.

Forrest, G.C. (1983) Mourning perinatal death. In: *Parent–Baby Attachment in Premature Infants* (eds. J.A. Davis, M.M.P. Richards & N.R. Roberton). Croom Helm, Beckenham.

Fox, P. (1988) Scars of the newborn caused by intensive care. *Neonatal Nurses Association Newsletter*, Autumn, 34–6.

Franck, L.S. (1986) A new method to quantitatively describe pain behavior in infants. *Nursing Research*, **35**, 28–31.

Franck, L.S. (1989) Pain in the non-verbal patient: advocating for the critically ill neonate. *Pediatric Nursing*, **15**(1), 65–8, 90.

Franck, L. & Vilardi, J. (1995) Assessment and management of opioid withdrawal in ill neonates. *Neonatal Network*, **14**(2), 39–45.

Freud, S. (1965) *A General Introduction of Psychoanalysis* (translated by J. Riviere). Washington Square Press, New York. (Originally published 1920.)

Furman, E. (1976) Comment in: *Maternal–Infant Bonding* (eds M.M. Klaus & J.H. Kennell). C.V. Mosby, St Louis.

Gale, G., Franck, L.S. & Lund, C. (1993) Skin-to-skin (Kangaroo) holding of the intubated premature infant. *Neonatal Network*, **12**(6), 49–57.

Garcia, A.P. & White-Traut, R.C. (1993) Preterm infants' responses to taste/smell and tactile stimulation during an apnoeic episode. *Journal of Pediatric Nursing*, **8**, 245–52.

Gauntlett, I.S. (1987) Analgesia in the neonate. *British Journal of Hospital Medicine*, June, 518–19.

Gaussen, T. & Hubley, P. (1987) Babies in special care: some developmental implications of adult–infant interactions. *Association for Child Psychiatry Newsletter*, **9**(4), 15–20.

Gauvain-Piquard, A. (1987) Comment reconnaître la douleur d'un enfant. *Revue de l'Infirmière*, **15**, 19–24.

Gauvain-Piquard, A., Rodary, C. & Lemerle, J. (1988) *L'Atonie Psychomotrice: Signe Majeur de Douleur Chez l'Enfant de Moins de Six Ans.*, pp. 249–52. Journées Parisiennes de Pédiatrie, Flammarion Médécine Sciences, Paris.

Gauvain-Piquard, A. (1989a) *La Douleur et le Bébé. Psychopathologie du Bébé* (eds S. Lebovici & F. Weil-Halperin) PUF of Paris.

Gauvain-Piquard, A. (1989b) *The Gustave-Roussy Child Pain Scale* (Douleur Enfant Gustave-Roussy – DEGR). Unité de psychiatrie et d'oncologie, Institut Gustave-Roussy, Villejuif, Paris.

Giannakoulopoulos, X., Sepulveda, W., Kouris, P., Glover, V., Fisk, N.M. (1994) Fetal plasma cortisol and β-endorphin response to intrauterine needling. *Lancet*, **344**, July 9, 77–81.

Glass, P., Avery, G.B., Kolinjavadi, N., Subramanian, S., Keys, M.P., Sostek, A.M. & Friendly, D.S. (1985) Effect of bright light in the hospital nursery on the incidence of retinopathy of prematurity. *New England Journal of Medicine*, **7**(313), 401–404.

Goble, P. (1993) *Beyond the Ridge*. Aladdin Books, Macmillan Publishing Company, New York.

Gordon, M. & Montgomery L.A. (1996) Minimizing epidermal stripping in the very low birth weight infant: integrating research and practice to affect infant outcome. *Neonatal Network*, **15**(1), 37–44.

Goren, S., Art, M. & Wu, P.K. (1975) Visual following and pattern discrimination of face-like stimuli by newborn infants. *Pediatrics*, **56**, 544.

Gorski, P.A. (1983) Premature infant behaviour and physiological responses to caregiving interventions in the intensive care nursery. In: *Frontiers of Infant Psychiatry* (eds J.D. Call, E. Galenson & R.L. Tyson), pp. 256–62. Basic Books, New York.

Gottfried, A.W., Hodgman, JE. & Brown, K.W. (1984) How intensive is newborn intensive care? An environmental analysis. *Pediatrics*, **74**, 292–4.

Gottlieb, G. (1971) Ontogenesis of sensory functioning in birds and mammals. In: *The Biopsychology of Development* (eds E. Tobach, L.R. Aronson & E. Shaw). Academic Press, New York.

Graham, F.K., Matarazzo, R.G. & Caldwell, B.M. (1956) Behavioral differences between normal and traumatised newborns: standardization, reliability and validity. In: *Psychological Monographs: General and Applied* (ed. H.S. Conrad), Vol. 70, pp. 1–33. The American Psychological Association, Washington DC.

Greeley, W.J., Boyd III, J.L. & Kern, F.H. (1993) Pharmacokinetics of analgesic drugs. In: *Pain in Neonates*. Pain Research and Clinical Management, Vol. 5 (eds K.J.S. Anand & P.J. McGrath). Elsevier, Amsterdam.

Greenacre, P. (1953) *Trauma, Growth and Personality*. Hogarth Press, London.

Greenough, A. & Greenall, F. (1988) Patient triggered ventilation in premature neonates. *Archives of Disease in Childhood*, **63**, 77–8.

Grossman, R.G. & Lawhon, G. (1993) Individualized supportive care to reduce pain and stress. In: *Pain in Neonates*. Pain Research and Clinical Management, Vol. 5 (eds K.J.S. Anand & P.J. McGrath). Elsevier, Amsterdam.

Grunau, R.V.E. & Craig, K.D. (1987) Pain expression in neonates: facial action and cry. *Pain*, **28**, 395–410.

Grunau, R.V.E., Johnstone, C.C. & Craig, K.D. (1990) Neonatal facial and cry responses to invasive and non-invasive procedures. *Pain*, **42**, 295–305.

Hall, M.A., Smith, S.L., Perks, E.M. & Walton, P. (1992) Neonatal nurse practitioners – a view from perfidious Albion? *Archives of Disease in Childhood*, **67**, 458–62.

Hannon, K.M. (1993). Support can reduce the stress factor. *Professional Nurse*, **8**(8), 496–500.

Hansen, D.D. & Hickey, P.R. (1986) Anesthesia for hypoplastic left heart syndrome: use of high-dose fentanyl in 30 neonates. *Anesthesia and Analgesia*, **65**, 127–32.

Harpin, V.A.H. & Rutter, N. (1982) Development of emotional sweating in the newborn infant. *Archives of Disease in Childhood*, **57**, 691–5.

Harpin, V.A.H. & Rutter, N. (1983) Making heel-pricks less painful. *Archives of Disease in Childhood*, **58**(3), 226–8.

Harris, T.A. (1973) *I'm OK – You're OK*. Pan Books, London.

Hawthorne, J.T., Richards, M.P.M. & Callon, M. (1978) A study of parental visiting of babies in a special care unit. In: *Early Separation and Special Care Nurseries. Clinics in Developmental Medicine*, Spastics International Medical Publications/Heinemann Medical Books, London.

Hay, B. (1990) Forgotten fathers? *BLINK (Blisslink newsletter)*, **2**, autumn/winter, 1, 4.

Henshall, W.R. (1972) Intrauterine sound levels. *American Journal of Obstetrics and Gynaecology*, **112**, 576–8.

Herzog, J. (1983) A neonatal intensive care syndrome: a pain complex involving neuroplasticity and psychic trauma. In: *Frontiers in Infant Psychiatry* (eds J. Calls, E. Galenson & R. Tuson), pp. 291–300. Basic Books, New York.

Hindmarch, C. (1993) *On the Death of a Child.* Radcliffe Medical Press, Oxford.

Hodge, D. (1991) Endotracheal suctioning and the infant: a nursing care protocol to decrease complications. *Neonatal Network,* **9**(5), 7–15.

Howell, S.H., Luna, M.L. & Miaskowski, C.A. (1985) Nonpharmacological therapies. In: *Pain. Nursing Now* series, Springfield, Corporation, Springhouse, Pennsylvania.

Hughes, B. & Hughes, E. (1993) Extra special care: a parent's eye view of a neonatal unit. *Child Health,* June/July, 29–32.

Huteau, M. (1988) Travail de recherche sur les sons et les prématurés. *Soins Gynécologie, Obstétrique, Puériculture, Pédiatrie,* **84**, 11–20.

Hutt, S.J. (1973) Auditory discrimination at birth. In: *Early Human Development* (eds S.J. Hutt & C. Hutt). Oxford University Press, Oxford.

Izard, C.E. & Bucchler, S. (1979) *Emotions in Personality and Psychopathology.* Plenum Press, New York.

Jacques, N.C.S., Hawthorne Amick, J.T. & Richards, M.P.M. (1983) Parents and the support they need. In: *Parent–Baby Attachment in Premature Infants* (eds J.A. Davis, M.P.M. Richards & N.R.C. Roberton). Croom Helm, Beckenham.

Jay, S.S. (1982) The effects of gentle human touch on mechanically ventilated very-short-gestation infants. *Maternal–Child Nursing Journal,* **11**, 199–256.

Johnston, C.C. & Strada, M.E. (1986) Acute pain response in infants: a multidimensional description. *Pain,* **24**, 28–31.

Jolly, H. (1975) *Book of Child Care.* George Allen & Unwin, London.

Kaminsky, J. & Hall, W. (1996) The effect of soothing music on neonatal behavioral states in the hospital newborn nursery. *Neonatal Network,* **15**(1), 45–54.

Kaplan, D.M. & Mason, E.A. (1960) Maternal reactions to premature birth viewed as an acute emotional disorder. *American Journal of Orthopsychiatry,* **30**(3), 539–52.

Kay, B. (1973) Neuroleptanesthesia for neonates and infants. *Anesthesia and Analgesia,* **52**(6), 970–973.

Kaye, K. (1982) *The Mental and Social Life of Babies.* University Press, London.

Kimble, D.L. (1991) Neonatal death: a descriptive study of fathers' experiences. *Neonatal Network,* **9**(8), 45–50.

Klaus, M.H. & Kennell, J.H. (1976) *Maternal–Infant Bonding.* C.V. Mosby, St. Louis.

Kleiber, C. (1986) Clinical implications of deep and shallow suctioning in neonatal patients. *Focus on Critical Care,* **13**(4), 36–9.

Kohner, N. & Henley, A. (1991) *When a Baby Dies.* Pandora Press, London.

Korones, S.B. (1976) Disturbance and infants' rest. In: *Report of 69th Ross Conference on Pediatric Research* (ed. T.D. Moore). Ross Laboratories, Columbus, Ohio.

Kraemer, L.I. & Pierpont, M.E. (1976) Rocking waterbeds and auditory stimuli to enhance growth of preterm infants: preliminary report. *Journal of Pediatrics,* **88**.

Kuhn, C.M., Schanberg, S.M., Field, T., Symanski, R., Zimerman, E., Scafidi, F. & Roberts J. (1991) Tactile-kinesthetic stimulation effects on sympathetic and adrenocortical function in preterm infants. *Journal of Pediatrics,* **119**, 434–40.

Kuhse, H. & Singer, P. (1985) Handicapped babies: a right to live? *Nursing Mirror*, **160**(8), 17–20.

Lagencrantz, H., Nilsson, F., Redham, I. & Hjemdal, P. (1986) Plasma catecholamines following nursing procedures in a neonatal ward. *Early Human Development*, **14** 61–5.

Lang, S. (1995) Alternative and supplementary methods of infant feeding: direct expression, cup-feeding, nursing supplementer, bottle-feeding, syringes and droppers. *The Neonatal Nurses' Yearbook*, 40–47.

Lassort, F., Kremer, C. & Rousseau, F. (1988) Evaluation des effets de l'enveloppe sonore. *Soins Gynécologie, Obstétrique, Puériculture, Pediatrice*, **84**, 21–6.

Lawhon, G. (1986) Management of stress in premature infants. *Perinatal/Neonatal Nursing* (ed. D.J. Angelini, D.J.). Blackwell, London.

Lawrence, J., Alcock, D., McGrath, P., Kay, J., MacMurray, S.B. & Dulberg, C. (1993) The development of a tool to assess neonatal pain. *Neonatal Network*, **12**(6), 59–66.

Lester, B.M. & Zeskind, P.S. (1982) A behavioral perspective on crying in early infancy. In: *Theory and Research in Behavioral Pediatrics*, Vol. I (eds H.E. Fitzgerald, B.M. Lester & M. Yogman). Plenum Publishing, New York.

Levene, M.I. & Quinn, M.W. (1992) Use of sedative and muscle relaxants in newborn babies receiving mechanical ventilation. *Archives of Disease in Childhood*, **67**, 870–873.

Lindemann, E. (1944) Symptomatology and management of acute grief. *American Journal of Psychiatry*, **101**, 141–8.

Long, G.J., Lucey, J.F. & Philip, A.G.S. (1980) Noise and hypoxaemia in the intensive care nursery. *Pediatrics*, **65**, 143–5.

Lotas, M.J. (1992) Effects of light and sound in the neonatal intensive care environment on the low-birth-weight infant. Nurses' Association of the American College of Obstetricians and Gynecologists. *Clinical Issues in Perinatal and Women's Health Nursing*, **3**(1), 34–44.

Lowe, G.R. (1972) *The Growth of Personality*. Penguin Books, London.

Ludman, L., Lansdown, R. & Spitz, L. (1989) Factors associated with developmental progress of full term neonates who required intensive care. *Archives of Disease in Childhood*, **64**, 333–7.

Lund, C., Kuller, J.M., Tobin, C., Lefrak, L. & Franck, L.S. (1986) Evaluation of a pectin-based barrier under tape to protect neonatal skin. *Journal of Obstetric, Gynocologic and Neonatal Nursing*, **15**(1), 39–44.

McCaffery, M. & Beebe, A. (1989) *Pain: Clinical Manual for Nursing Practice*. C.V. Mosby, St. Louis.

McFarlane, Baroness & Castledine, G. (1982) *A Guide to the Practice of Nursing using the Nursing Process*. C.V. Mosby, New York.

McGrath, P.J. (1993) Research design and research ethics. In: *Pain in Neonates*. Pain Research and Clinical Management, Vol. 5 (eds K.J.S. Anand & P.J. McGrath). Elsevier, Amsterdam.

McGrath, P. & Unruh, A. (1987) *Pain in Children and Adolescents*. Elsevier, Amsterdam.

McGraw, M.B. (1941) Neural maturation as exemplified in the changing reactions of the infant to pin prick. *Child Development*, **12**, 31–42.

McIlwain, H. (1970) Metabolic adaptation in the brain. *Nature*, **226**, 803–806.

McIntosh, N. (1983) The monitoring of critically ill neonates. *Journal of Medical Engineering and Technology*, **7**(3), 121–9.

McKee, C.M., Priest, P., Ginzler, M. & Black, N.A. (1991) How can the work of junior paeditricians be reduced? *Archives of Disease in Childhood*, **66**, 1085–89.

Mann, N., Haddon, R., Stokes, L. *et al.* (1986) Effect of night and day on preterm infants in a newborn nursery: randomized trial. *British Medical Journal*, **293**, 1265–7.

Marshall, R.E., Porter, F.L., Rogers, A.G., Moore, J.A., Anderson, B. & Boxerman, S.B. (1982) Circumcision II. Effects upon mother–infant interaction. *Early Human Development*, **7**, 367–74.

Maunuksela, E.-L. & Korpela, R. (1986) Double blind evaluation of a lignocaine-prilocaine cream (EMLA) in children. *British Journal of Anaesthesiology*, **58**, 1242–5.

Maury, C. (1988) Prolégomènes à la thérapie sonore dans le service des prématurés. *Soins Gynécologie, Obstétrique, Puériculture, Pédiatrie*, **84**, 9–10.

Melzack, R. & Wall, P. (1988) *The Challenge of Pain*, 3rd edn. Penguin Books, London.

Mersky, H. (1986) Classification of chronic pain: descriptions of chronic pain syndromes and definitions of pain items. *Pain*, Supplement 3, 51–225. Elsevier, Amsterdam.

Messer, D., Harris, G. & St. James-Roberts, I. (1993) An overview of infant crying, feeding and sleeping problems. In: *Infant Crying, Feeding and Sleeping* (eds I. St. James-Roberts, G. Harris & D. Messer). Harvester Wheatsheaf, Hemel Hempstead.

Michaëlsson, M., Riesenfeld, T. & Sagren, A. (1992) High noise levels in incubators can be reduced. *Acta Paediatrica*, **81**(10), 843–4.

Michelsson, A-L., Jarvenpaa, A-L. & Rinne, A. (1983) Sound spectographic analysis of pain cry in preterm infants. *Early Human Development*, **8**, 141–9.

Minde, K. & Minde, R. (1986) *Infant Psychiatry: An Introductory Textbook*. Sage Publications, Beverly Hills.

Mitchell, A. (1996) Thermal monitoring of patients in NICU. *Journal of Neonatal Nursing*, **2**(2), central insert.

Mok, Q., Bass, C.A., Ducker, D.A. & McIntosh, N. (1991) Temperature instability during nursing procedures in preterm neonates. *Archives of Disease in Childhood*, **66**, 783–6.

Monset-Couchard, M., de Bethman, O., Radranyi-Bouvet, M.F., Papin, C., Bordariev, C. & Relier, J.P. (1988) Neurodevelopmental outcome in cystic periventricular leukomalacia. *Neuropediatrics*, **19**, 124–31.

Moore, P. (1995) *Born Too Early*. Thorsons (imprint of HarperCollins Publishers), London.

Morris, M. (1994) Neonatal care today. In: *Neonatal Nursing* (eds D. Crawford & M. Morris). Chapman & Hall, London.

Munsinger, H. (1970) Light detection and pattern recognition: some comments on the growth of visual sensation and perception. In: *Lifespan Developmental*

Psychology: Research and Theory (eds. L.R. Goulet & P.B. Bultes), pp. 227–46. Academy Press, New York.

Murdoch, D.R. & Darlow, B.A. (1984) Handling during neonatal intensive care. *Archives of Disease in Childhood*, **59**, 957–61.

Murooka, H., Kove, Y. & Suda, N. (1976) Analysis of inter-uterine sounds and their tranquillising effects on the newborn infant. *Journal de Gynécologie, Obstétrique et Biologie de la Reproduction*, **5**(3), 367–76.

Mussen, P.H., Conger, J.J., Kagan, J. & Huston, A.C. (1984) *Child Development and Personality*. Harper International Edition, Harper & Row, New York.

Nathan, P. (1988) *The Nervous System*, 3rd ed. Oxford University Press, Oxford.

Neumann, E. (1973) *The Child: Structure and Dynamics of the Nascent Personality*. Harper & Row, New York.

Norton, J.J. (1988) After effects of morphine and fentanyl analgesia: a retrospective study. *Neonatal Network*, **7**, 25–8.

Oberklaid, F., Sewell, J., Sanson, A. & Prior, M. (1991) Temperament and behavior of preterm infants: a six-year follow-up. *Pediatrics*, **87**(6), 854–61.

Osterweis, M., Solomon, F. & Green, M. (1984) *Bereavement: Reactions, Consequences and Care*. National Academy Press, Washington.

Owens, M.E. (1984) Pain in infancy: conceptual and methodological issues. *Pain*, **20**, 213–30.

Pape, K.E. & Wigglesworth, J.S. (1979) Hemorrhage, ischaemia and the perinatal brain. *Clinics in Developmental Medicine*, No. 69/70. J.B. Lippincott, Philadelphia.

Papoušek, H. & Papoušek, M. (1983) Interactional failures, their origins and significance in infant psychiatry. In: *Frontiers of Infant Psychiatry* (eds J.D. Call, E. Galensen & R.L. Tyson), pp. 31–7. Basic Books, New York.

Patton Dunbar, C. (1995) Quality within neonatal nursing: getting the skill mix balance right. *Journal of Neonatal Nursing*, **1**(5), 19–23.

Perlman, J.M. & Volpe, J.J. (1983) Suctioning in the preterm infant: effects on cerebral blood flow velocity, intracranial pressure and arterial blood pressure. *Pediatrics*, **65**, 143–5.

Piaget, J. (1970) Piaget's theory. In: *Carmichael's Manual of Child Psychology* (ed P.H. Mussen), Vol. 1, 3rd edn. John Wiley, New York.

Pidcock, F.S., Graziani, L.J., Stanley, C., Mitchell, D.G. & Merton, D. (1990) Neurosonographic features of periventricular echodensities associated with cerebral palsy in preterm infants. *Journal of Pediatrics*, **116**, 417–22.

Prugh, D.G., Jordan, K., Beresford, T.P., Marshall, M.D., Black, D. & Wood, D. (1983) Hypertrophic pyloric stenosis in infancy: innate and experimental factors. In: *Frontiers of Infant Psychiatry* (eds J.D. Call, E. Galenson & R.L. Tyson), pp. 301–323. Basic Books, New York.

Reber, A. (1985) *Dictionary of Psychology*. Penguin Books, London.

Redman, C. (1993) Putting the family back in control: neonatal intensive care units and the emotional needs of families. *Child Health*, **1**(3), 112–16.

Redshaw, M. & Harris, A. (1995) Quality and quantity: staffing and skill mix in neonatal care. *Nursing Times*, **91**(27), 29–31.

Richards, M.P.M. (1978) Effects on development of medical interventions and the separation of newborns from their parents. *The First Year of Life* (eds. D. Shaffer & J. Dunn). John Wiley, London.

Richards, M.P.M. (1983) Parent–child relationships. In: *Parent-Baby Attachment in Premature Infants* (eds J.A. Davies, M.P.M. Richards & N.R.C. Roberton). Croom Helm, Beckenham.

Roberton, N.R.C. (1986) *A Manual of Neonatal Intensive Care*, 2nd edn. Edward Arnold, London.

Rogers, M. (1980) Nursing: a science of unitary man. In: *Conceptual Models for Nursing Practice* (eds J. Riehl & C. Roy). Appleton–Century–Crofts, New York.

Roper, N. (1976) A model of nursing and nurseology. *Journal of Advanced Nursing*, **1**(3), 219–27.

Rosenblith, J.F. (1961) The Modified Graham Behavior Test for Neonates: test–retest reliability, normative data, and hypotheses for future work. *Biology of the Neonate*, **3**, 174–92.

Rowe, T.S., Keats, J.N. & Morgan, J. (1987) A new approach to the management of extravasation injury in neonates. *Pharmaceutical Journal*, **14**.

Rubel, E.E. (1985) Auditory system development. In: *Measurement of Audition and Vision in the First Year of Post Natal Life: A Methodological Overview* (eds G. Gottlieb & N.A. Krasnegor), pp. 53–89. Ablex, Norwood, New Jersey.

Rushton, C. (1986) Promoting normal growth and development in the hospital environment. *Neonatal Network*, **4**(6), 21–30.

Saling, A. (1985) *Gherasche in utero*. Demonstration tape. Institut für Perinatale Medizin, Berlin.

Sarnat, H.B. (1978) Olfactory reflexes in the newborn infant. *Journal of Pediatrics*, **92**, 624–6.

Sayre-Adams, J. (1994) Therapeutic Touch: a nursing function. *Nursing Standard*, **8**(17), 25–8.

Scafidi, F., Field, T., Schanberg, S., Bauer, C., Vega-Lahr, N. & Garcia, R. (1986) Effects of tactile kinesthetic stimulation on the clinical course and sleep/wake behavior of preterm neonates. *Infant Behavior and Development*, **9**, 91–105.

Schlomann, P. (1992) Ethical considerations of aggressive care of very low birth weight infants. *Neonatal Network*, **11**(4), 31–6.

Schraeder, B. (1986) Developmental progress of very low birth weight infants during the first year of life. *Nursing Research*, **35**(4), 237–42.

Seligmann, M. (1975) *Helplessness. On Depression, Development and Death*. W.H. Freeman, Oxford.

Shellabarger, S.G. & Thompson, T.L. (1993) The critical times: meeting parental communication needs throughout the NICU experience. *Neonatal Network*, 12 March(2), 39–44.

Shorten, D.C., Byrne, P.J. & Jones, R.L. (1991) Infant responses to saline instillation and endotracheal suctioning. *Neonatal Nursing*, **20**(6), 464–9.

Sofaer, B. (1985) Pain management through nurse education. In: *Perspectives on Pain*. (ed. L.S. Copp). Churchill Livingstone, New York.

Soulé, M. (1986) Les aspects psychologiques de la réanimation d'un nouveau né. *Archives Françaises de Pédiatrie*, **43**(1), 555–7.

Sparshott, M.M. (1989a) Pain and the Special Care Baby Unit. *Nursing Times*, **85**, 61–4.

Sparshott, M.M. (1989b) Minimising discomfort of sick newborns. *Nursing Times*, **85**(42), 39–42.

Sparshott, M.M. (1989c) *This is Your Baby: How to understand your baby and what to do to help him grow.* Printed for the NICU, Derriford Hospital, Plymouth.

Sparshott, M.M. (1990) The human touch. *Paediatric Nursing*, **2**(5), 8–10.

Sparshott, M.M. (1991a) Maintaining skin integrity. *Paediatric Nursing*, **3**(2), 12–13.

Sparshott, M.M. (1991b) Psychological function of the skin. *Paediatric Nursing*, **3**(3), 22–3.

Sparshott, M.M. (1991c) Creating a home for babies in hospital. *Paediatric Nursing*, **3**(8), 20–22.

Sparshott, M.M. (1993) Comment soutenir les parents des enfants prématurés: experience anglaise. In: *VIIes Journées des Soins en Pédiatrie, abstract: Le Stress*, Nantes, 10–12 Juin.

Sparshott, M.M. (1994) Nursing care of a baby in pain and discomfort. In: *Neonatal Nursing* (eds D. Crawford & M. Morris). Chapman & Hall, London.

Sparshott, M.M. (1995a) The 'sound' – of neonatal nursing care. *Journal of Neonatal Nursing*, **1**(2), 7–9.

Sparshott, M.M. (1995b) Assessing the behaviour of the newborn infant. *Paediatric Nursing*, **7**(7), 14–16, 36.

Sparshott, M.M. (1996) The development of a clinical distress scale for ventilated newborn infants: identification of pain and distress based on validated behavioural scores. *Journal of Neonatal Nursing*, **2**(2), 5–11.

Squire, L.R. (1986) Mechanisms of memory. *Science*, **232**, 1612–19.

Sroufe, L.A. (1979) Socioemotional development. In: *Handbook of Infant Development* (ed J.D. Osofsky). John Wiley, New York.

Stickney, D. (1984) *Water Bugs and Dragonflies.* The Pilgrim Press, Mowbray, London.

Strauch, C., Brandt, S. & Edwards-Beckett, J. (1993) Implementation of a quiet hour: effect on noise levels and infant sleep states. *Neonatal Network*, **12**(2), 31–5.

Third Maternity Services Advisory Committee Report (1985) *Staffing for Postnatal and Neonatal Care*, Chapter 8, 43–47.

Tribotti, S.J. & Stein, M. (1992) From research to clinical practice: implementing the NIDCAP. *Neonatal Network*, **11**(2), 35–40.

Turrill, S. (1992) Supported positioning in intensive care. *Paediatric Nursing*, May, 24–7.

Updike, C., Schmidt, R.E., Cahoon, J. & Miller, M. (1986) Positional support for premature infants. *The American Journal of Occupational Therapy*, **40**(10), 712–15.

Uvnas-Möberg, K., Widstrom, A.M., Marchini, G. & Winberg, J. (1987) Release of GI hormones in mother and infant by sensory stimulation. *Acta Paediatrica Scandinavica*, **76**, 851–60.

VandenBerg, K.A. (1995) Behaviorally supportive care for the extremely premature infant. In: *Care of the 24–25 week gestational age infant (small baby protocol)* (eds L.P. Gunderson & C. Kenner). Neonatal Network, Petaluma, California.

VandenBerg, K.A. (1996) Developmental care: is it working? *Neonatal Network*, **15**(1), 67–9.

Van der Bor, M., Guit, G.L., Schreuder, A.M., Wondergem, J. & Vielroye, G.J. (1989) Early detection of delayed myelination in preterm infants. *Pediatrics*, **84**, 407–11.

Varley, S. (1985) *Badger's Parting Gifts*. Andersen Press, London.

Vine, T. (1995) The father's role on the neonatal unit. *Journal of Neonatal Nursing*, **1**(2), 23–7.

Voyer, M. (1986) Ethique et handicap en réanimation: l'accompagnement lors de la mort d'un enfant. *Archives Française de la Pédiatrie*, **43**(1), 575–8.

Wachter-Shikora, N.L. (1981) Pain theories and their relevance to the pediatric population. In: *Issues in Comprehensive Pediatric Nursing*, Vol. 5. Hemisphere Publishing Corporation, San Francisco.

Walker, C.H.M. (1982) Neonatal intensive care and stress. *Archives of Disease in Childhood*, **57**, 85 8.

Walker, P. (1995) *Baby Massage*. Judy Piatkus (Publishers), London.

Washington, J., Minde, K. & Goldberg, S. (1986) Temperament in preterm infants: style and stability. *Journal of the American Academy of Child Psychiatry*, **25**, 493–502.

Wasunna, A. & Whitelaw, A.G.L. (1987) Pulse oximetry in preterm infants. *Archives of Disease in Childhood*, **62**, 957–71.

Weibley, T.T., Adamson, N., Clinkscales, N., Curran, J. & Bramson, R. (1987) Gavage tube insertion in the premature infant. *Maternal Child Nursing Journal*, **12**, 24–7.

White-Traut, R.C. & Goldman, M.B.C. (1988) Premature infant massage: is it safe? *Pediatric Nursing*, **14**(4), 285–9.

White-Traut, R.C., Nelson, M.N., Silvestri, J., Patel,M. & Kilgallon, D. (1993) Patterns of physiological and behavioral response of immediate care preterm infants to intervention. *Pediatric Nursing*, **19**, 625–9.

White-Traut, R.C., Nelson, M.N., Burns, K. & Cunningham, N. (1994) Environmental influences on the developing premature infant: theoretical issues and applications to practice. *Journal of Obstetric, Gynocologic and Neonatal Nursing*, **23**(5), 393–400.

Whitelaw, A. (1986) Skin-to-skin contact in the care of very low birth weight babies. *Maternal and Child Health*, July, 242–6.

Whitelaw, A. & Valman, B. (1980) Taking blood and putting up a drip in young children. *British Medical Journal*, **281** (6240), 602–604.

Whitworth, C.M. & Topping, A. (1996) The interface between policy, quality and research: an action research approach to promote successful breastfeeding. *Journal of Neonatal Nursing*, **2**(2), 20–23.

Widmayer, S. & Field, T. (1980) Effects of Brazelton demonstrations on early interactions of preterm infants and their teenage mothers. *Infant Behavior and Development*, **3**, 78–89.

Williamson, P.S. & Williamson, M.L. (1983) Physiological stress reduction by a local anaesthetic during newborn circumcision. *Pediatrics*, **71**(1), 360–400.

Wilson, G., Hughes, G., Rennie, J. & Morley, C. (1992) Evaluation of two endotracheal suction regimes in babies ventilated for respiratory distress syndrome. *Neonatal Network*, **11**(7), 43–4.

Winnicott, D.W. (1957) *The Child and the Family*. Tavistock Publications, London.

Winnicott, D.W. (1965) The theory of parent–infant relationship. In: *The Maturational Processes and the Facilitating Environment*. Hogarth Press, London.

Winnicott, D.W. (1975) *Through Paediatrics to Psychoanalysis*. Hogarth Press, London.

Wolff, P.H. (1966) *The Causes, Controls and Organization of Behaviour in the Neonate*. International University Press, New York.

Wolff, P.H. (1969) The natural history of crying and other vocalizations in early infancy. *Determinants of Infant Behaviour*, **4**, 81–115.

Wolke, D. (1987) Environmental and developmental neonatology. *Journal of Reproductive and Infant Psychiatry*, **5**, 17–42.

Wynnejones, P. (1985) *Children, Death and Bereavement*. Scripture Union, Trinity Press, Worcester.

Yaster, M. (1987) The dose response of fentanyl in neonatal anesthesia. *Anesthesiology*, **66**, 433–55.

Young, J. (1995) To help or hinder: endotracheal suction and the intubated neonate. *Journal of Neonatal Nursing*, **1**(4), 23–8.

Zaiwalla, Z. & Stein, A. (1993) The physiology of sleep in infants and young children. In: *Infant Crying, Feeding and Sleeping* (eds I. St. James-Roberts, G. Harris & D. Messer). Harvester Wheatsheaf, Hemel Hempstead.

Index